INTERNATIONAL SYMPOSIA ON ALCOHOL AND DRUG ADDICTION

VOLUMES IN THIS SERIES

BIOLOGICAL AND BEHAVIOURAL APPROACHES TO DRUG DEPENDENCE
H. D. Cappell and A. E. Le Blanc

SOCIAL ASPECTS OF THE MEDICAL USE OF PSYCHOTROPIC DRUGS
R. Cooperstock

RESEARCH ON METHODS AND PROGRAMS OF DRUG EDUCATION
M. Goodstadt

ALCOHOLIC LIVER PATHOLOGY
J. M. Khanna, Y. Israel and H. Kalant

STREET DRUG ANALYSIS AND ITS SOCIAL AND CLINICAL IMPLICATIONS
J. A. Marshman

EXPERIMENTATION IN CONTROLLED ENVIRONMENT: ITS IMPLICATIONS FOR ECONOMIC BEHAVIOUR AND SOCIAL POLICY MAKING
C. G. Miles

EFFECTS OF CHRONIC USE OF ALCOHOL AND OTHER PSYCHOACTIVE DRUGS ON CEREBRAL FUNCTION
J. G. Rankin

CLINICAL PHARMACOLOGY AND TOXICOLOGY OF PSYCHOACTIVE DRUGS
E. M. Sellers

Available from: Marketing Services,
Addiction Research Foundation,
33 Russell Street,
Toronto, Ontario M5S 2S1.

ALCOHOL, DRUGS AND BRAIN DAMAGE

Proceedings of a Symposium: Effects of Chronic Use of Alcohol and other Psychoactive Drugs on Cerebral Function

Edited by JAMES G. RANKIN

General Editor: S. L. LAMBERT

ALCOHOLISM AND DRUG
ADDICTION RESEARCH FOUNDATION
OF ONTARIO
TORONTO • CANADA

All the papers in this series were presented at the International Symposia on Alcohol and Drug Research co-sponsored by the Department of National Health and Welfare, Ottawa, Canada, and the Alcoholism and Drug Addiction Research Foundation, Toronto, Canada, in association with the International Council on Alcohol and Addictions, Lausanne, Switzerland.

October, 1973

International Standard Book Number: 0-88868-009-0.

1975

Printed in Canada – House of Lind

Contents

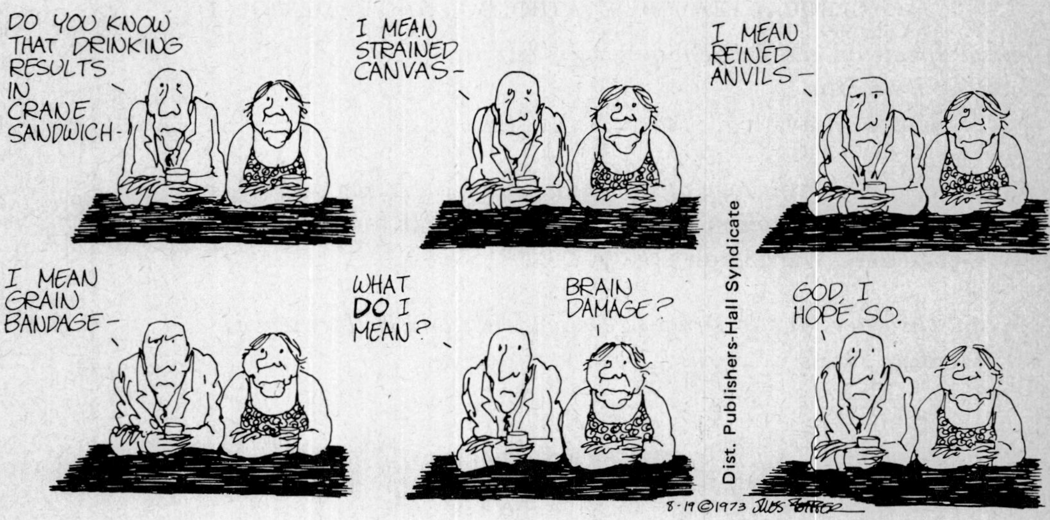
DO YOU KNOW THAT DRINKING RESULTS IN CRANE SANDWICH-
I MEAN STRAINED CANVAS-
I MEAN REINED ANVILS-
I MEAN GRAIN BANDAGE-
WHAT DO I MEAN?
BRAIN DAMAGE?
GOD, I HOPE SO.
Dist. Publishers-Hall Syndicate
8-19 ©1973

As is so often the case, it is the cartoonist who, as a perceptive observer, makes critical comments on important aspects of human behaviour and their consequences, which may often be largely unrecognized, neglected or ignored by those who should be most concerned. In this context Jules Feiffer drew attention to the problem of alcohol-related brain damage in his cartoon published in August 1973, two months before this symposium was held. He skilfully depicts the distressing, pitiful problem of alcoholic dementia, a problem which has attracted little medical interest and concern, relative to its prevalence and serious significance. Visual commentaries such as Feiffer's should be recognized as part of a continuum of social commentary about problems of alcohol use by cartoonists and other artists over the centuries, a commentary which to varying degrees has been influential in focusing attention on these problems and assisting in their resolution.

Introduction

Clinically manifest brain damage, in its various forms, associated with prolonged hazardous consumption of alcohol is about as common as alcoholic cirrhosis, whilst subclinical, reversible brain damage manifested by disturbances of psychometric tests has a prevalence of the same order of magnitude as subclinical, acute, reversible alcoholic liver disease. Indeed it is to be expected that amongst those who drink hazardously there will be found a spectrum of cerebral function ranging from complete normality to utter derangement, a spectrum which may be either obscured or unrecognized because of the fairly constant superimposition of disturbances of cerebral function caused by the continuing acute effects of alcohol or intermittent withdrawal in such individuals.

While there is substantial agreement that chronic hazardous consumption of alcohol is associated with brain damage, aetiology is a matter of debate. On the one hand, it is clear that in the alcoholic individual thiamine deficiency alone can cause irreversible changes in the diencephalon, brainstem and cerebellum, changes that are clinically manifested by the Wernicke-Korsakoff syndrome and alcoholic cerebellar disease respectively. What is unclear is whether alcohol alone can produce neuronal injury and death, as well as to what extent other factors may be important in either precipitating or aggravating brain damage due to alcohol and/or thiamine deficiency. Examples would include trauma, anoxia, and genetic inheritance. Indeed, in the individual demented alcoholic patient, it is quite possible, even probable, that over the years a series of factors may have contributed, each in its own way, to a cumulative destruction of neurones, a pathological process that is ultimately clinically manifested when the degree of damage exceeds the ability of the brain to adapt.

Whether the chronic use of psychoactive substances other than alcohol produces significant neuronal injury and death is a question with no clear answer, and often a subject of heated debate in which positions taken are more often based on beliefs than on analysis of scientific evidence.

If we know so little about the cerebral effects of the chronic use of drugs other than alcohol, then we certainly know even less about the potential consequences to the brain from the chronic hazardous use of alcohol in combination with other psychoactive substances. This latter pattern of use is becoming increasingly common and may be one which we ultimately come to recognize as leading to an increased prevalence and severity of brain damage over and above that which would have occurred had the hazardous use been of alcohol or drugs alone.

Why should we be so concerned about brain damage associated with chronic alcohol or drug use? Reasons for concern can be examined from three perspectives: the individual with brain damage, current magnitude of the problem of alcohol and drug-related brain damage in Canada, and finally changing trends in that magnitude.

In the case of the individual patient with alcohol-related brain damage, the disturbance may be so severe that he or she is unable to function effectively as an independent being. In other patients, damage is less severe and yet clinically manifest; they almost invariably continue their alcohol consumption, despite all therapeutic efforts, and to the further detriment of their cerebral function. We must also consider the possibility that in some individuals subclinical brain damage may be a significant factor impairing their ability to reduce their intake or abstain from alcohol.

A reasonable, minimal estimate of the current number of individuals in Canada with alcohol-related brain damage is 18,000 *i.e.,* 5% of the alcoholic population. On the basis of changes in per capita consumption of alcohol use we can predict with reasonable confidence that the prevalence of alcohol-related brain damage has progressively increased since 1933 and probably doubled in the last 20 years. We can also predict that it will continue to increase until such time as some action brings about either a stabilization or reduction in per capita consumption.

The reasons why we still know so relatively little about brain damage associated with the chronic use of alcohol and other psychoactive substances are many. First, this does not appear to have been a subject that has attracted extensive, protracted research such as has been the case in alcoholic liver disease where much more progress has been made. Whether this deficit in research is mainly due to a lack of interest by neurological investigators in chronic problems of alcohol and drug dependence or whether it is related to inherent difficulties in carrying out research into chronic brain disease generally, is impossible to say, but certainly these do appear to be the two basic factors.

Difficulties of alcohol and drug-related brain damage research in man are posed by the relative inaccessibility of the human brain to direct study during life; the problems of studying a disease that probably has a combined subclinical and clinical course of 20 to 30 years; the great plasticity of cerebral function; the difficulties of assessing the significance of potential aetiological factors, particularly when there may have been a large temporal gap between the time when injury occurred and when it became clinically manifest; the need for appropriate, sensitive, easily administered, rapid, quantitative tests of brain function; and finally, the knowledge that whatever are the adverse consequences of chronic alcohol and drug use on cerebral function, they are being studied in individuals where the brain is also subject to other disease processes which are relatively common causes of dementia, as well as the normal process of cerebral ageing.

Many of these methodological difficulties in man could be overcome in the laboratory animal. However, to date, animal experimentation has not been extensively used to study the effects on brain function of chronic alcohol and other drug use, particularly in contrast to the number of studies which have led to considerable understanding of the acute effects of these agents.

This, then, is the background against which the present symposium was planned. The objective of the meeting was to examine the present state of knowledge about the effects of chronic use of alcohol and other psychoactive substances on cerebral function, particularly intellect, learning and memory, and to explore and if possible define, important research questions and needs.

One basic strategy of the meeting was to bring together scientists whose work was concentrated in the field of alcoholism and drug dependence with others working in areas of behaviour, cerebral function and disease unrelated to alcohol and drug use. In all, there were twenty-one participants – pharmacologists, psychologists, psychiatrists, neurologists and specialists in internal medicine – from Australia, England, Italy, Sweden, the United States and Canada. This group would have been unlikely to have met together under any other circumstances, yet it seemed possible that their individual contributions would potentially complement one another and in so doing yield a much clearer view and perspective of the subject under examination.

The second strategy was to structure the meeting and invite papers on specific aspects of the subject in the hope the composite of the resultant contributions would provide a systematic examination, as well as an overview and perspective, on the effects of chronic use of alcohol and other psychoactive substances on cerebral function. As might be expected, such an approach tended to give some authors greater difficulty than others because of the present inadequacy of knowledge on particular aspects; it was also likely to result in conflict with other aspects where available data were either conflicting or open to conflicting interpretation. The resultant eight papers were a composite of original research of the participants, literature reviews and speculation.

The topic and the papers stimulated an extensive discussion which ranged widely over aspects of alcoholism and drug dependence, and acute and chronic effects of psychoactive substances and brain damage. The following were identified as important research topics, needs or approaches: improvement in techniques to identify and measure sub-clinical or early clinical brain damage; clarification of the nature and basis of reversible abnormalities in psychological tests of cerebral function which are commonly observed in alcoholic patients; further studies of the natural history of brain damage associated with alcohol and drug use including a comparison of clinical features with brain pathology; much more extensive use of laboratory animals to determine the effects of chronic alcohol and drug use on the brain.

It was decided not to publish the total discussions. However, it is hoped that the eight papers being published will provide readers with a comprehensive review of the subject and in so doing, also stimulate ongoing interest and further research.

J.G.R.

Appreciation is expressed to all the Symposium contributors for their interest, efforts and enthusiasm; to Sylvia Lambert and Ruth Lamont for their hard work, assistance and tolerance; and to Jules Feiffer for permission to reproduce his cartoon commentary on alcoholic brain damage.

PARTICIPANTS

Dr. Peter Ashby	Division of Neurology Toronto Western Hospital Toronto, Canada
Professor J. Botwinick	Director of Aging and Development Program Department of Psychology Washington University St. Louis, Missouri, U.S.A.
Dr. Daniele Bovet	Professor of Pharmacology University of Sassari (Sardinia) Consiglio Naxionale delle Ricerche Rome, Italy
Dr. D. R. Crapper	Professor of Physiology Associate Professor of Medicine Staff Neurologist Toronto General Hospital Toronto, Ontario, Canada
Mr. Jan de Lint	Research Scientist Addiction Research Foundation Toronto, Canada
Dr. Pierre Dreyfus	Department of Neurology School of Medicine University of California Davis, California, U.S.A.
Dr. Myrddin Evans	Consultant in Psychiatry University Hospital of Wales, and Director of the Addiction Unit, Whitchurch Hospital Cardiff, Wales
Dr. Donald W. Goodwin	Professor Psychiatry Director, Washington University Addiction Research Center Washington University School of Medicine St. Louis, Missouri, U.S.A.
Dr. Lars-M. Gunne	Psychiatric Research Centre University of Uppsala Ulleraker Hospital Uppsala, Sweden
Dr. Shirley Y. Hill	Department of Psychiatry Washington University School of Medicine St. Louis, Missouri

Dr. Thomas Horvath	Department of Psychiatry Stanford University Medical Center Stanford, California, U.S.A.
Dr. Harold Kalant	Department of Pharmacology University of Toronto, and Biological Studies Department Addiction Research Foundation Toronto, Canada
Dr. S. George Laverty	Director, Addiction Studies Unit Kingston Psychiatric Hospital Kingston, Canada
Dr. Mary Ann Linseman	Research Scientist Addiction Research Foundation Toronto, Canada
Dr. Simone Radouco-Thomas	Department of Pharmacology Laval University Quebec City, Canada
Dr. V. Rakoff	Professor of Psychiatric Education Department of Psychiatry University of Toronto Toronto, Canada
Dr. James G. Rankin	Director and Head of Medicine Addiction Research Foundation Clinical Institute, and Associate Professor of Medicine University of Toronto
Dr. E. K. Warrington	Psychologist National Hospitals for Nervous Diseases Queen's Square London, England
Professor Bernard Weiss	Department of Radiation Biology and Biophysics University of Rochester School of Medicine and Dentistry Rochester, New York, U.S.A.
Dr. D. Adrian Wilkinson	Psychologist Addiction Research Foundation Toronto, Canada
Dr. Patricia Wilkinson	Department of Community Medicine St. Vincent's Hospital Melbourne, Australia

Clinical Spectrum and Epidemiological Features of Alcoholic Dementia

Thomas B. Horvath

INTRODUCTION

Chronic brain syndrome or dementia, that is, a progressive and largely irreversible impairment of intellectual function, memory and social behaviour is not an uncommon complication of alcoholism. Bonhoeffer in 1904 estimated its prevalence at 3% of all chronic alcoholics, and Pollock at 10% (1). The first admission rate of alcoholics with chronic brain disorders to California State hospitals in the 1950s was 7.5 per 100,000 of the general population. In Victoria, Australia, the admission rate of patients with alcoholic dementia to mental hospitals was 7 per 100,000 during the sixties. A health survey of 1000 alcoholics (2) in the same state revealed that 9% of these patients were demented.

It appears to have become common practice to label any demented alcoholic patient as suffering from Korsakoff's psychosis. It became apparent to the author, with increasing experience in a general hospital alcoholism clinic, that only a fraction of the demented patients showed the clear clinical features of Korsakoff's psychosis. The aim of the present paper is to review the spectrum of the manifestations of chronic brain syndrome in alcoholics, based on a search of the literature and a clinical study of 100 demented alcoholics seen at one clinic over a five-year period.

HISTORICAL BACKGROUND

Drunkenness is one of the few socially sanctioned forms of aberrant mentation and behaviour. The impairment of psychic and motor abilities is so striking that it has always been easy to extrapolate to a permanent loss of cerebral function as a consequence of chronic excessive drinking. In 1852, Magnus Huss was already able to refer to 56 monographs on the consequences of chronic inebriety published during the preceding 400 years (3). He systematized these old observations on the decline in physical and mental health of inveterate drinkers, and described such common abnormalities as dullness of thought and judgment, impairment of memory, hallucinations, deliria, melancholia, mania and anxiety. He recognized that the common pathway for the production of mental symptoms was the impairment of brain function, and a promising way of investigation was the pathological examination of the brain. While Sutton (4) and Canton (5) could only find nonspecific hyperaemia of the brain in cases of delirium tremens, Annan (6) described softening of the cortex and the thalamus in a case of "idiocy from intemperance".

Lawson (7) in 1879 also attributed many of the mental aberrations of alcoholics to brain disorders, associating the chronic conditions with cerebral degeneration. He noted not only a general dementia, but also a state resembling general paresis of the insane, and a peculiar state of "absolute loss of memory for recent events ..... with other mental functions well preserved". Anstie (8) in 1868 described the development of dementia in association with epilepsy, locomotor ataxia, and peripheral sensory loss in alcoholic patients. Bevan Lewis (9) in 1889 defined three forms of chronic alcoholic mental disturbances: "amnesic", "delusional" and "simple dementia". Maudsley (10) noted that the mental deterioration of these subjects consisted of a severely impaired memory, childish understanding, blunted moral sense and weak will power. If their drinking were not arrested, then a state of complete dementia supervened, with verbal incoherence, mental confusion, delusions and fantastic hallucinations.

In 1887 Korsakoff (11, 12) gave a description of a disturbance of psychic activities seen in association with multiple neuritis in alcoholic patients. It is worth noting that in this paper he described not only the characteristic memory loss but also clouding of consciousness, confusion and inconsistency of ideas, and irritable depression of mood. In a later article (13), describing 14 non-alcoholics, the clinical picture is restricted to what we now call Korsakoff's psychosis: loss of memory for recent events in the presence of otherwise normal mental capacity.

Bonhoeffer (14) was the first to recognize clearly the relation of Korsakoff's psychosis to a neuropathological syndrome described by Wernicke in 1881, which consisted of the association of ophthalmoplegia, ataxia and stupor with punctate haemorrhages around the third and fourth ventricles in the grey matter. While not all the patients with amnesia and midbrain neurological signs and peripheral neuropathy were alcoholics, Bonhoeffer classified Korsakoff's psychosis among the chronic alcoholic brain disorders.

Mott (15) in 1910 divided the alcoholic psychoses into two groups: those resulting from the direct or indirect action of alcohol on the previously healthy brain over a prolonged period of time, and those resulting from the action of alcohol on a potentially insane person. In the former group he recognized only two disorders: delirium tremens and Korsakoff's psychosis. Mott may be seen as the originator of the practice to label any confused and delirious alcoholic as suffering from delirium tremens and any deteriorated and demented drinker as having Korsakoff's psychosis.

CLASSIFICATION

The early classifications of alcoholic mental disorders were based entirely on the phenomenology of these conditions (Bonhoeffer (16); Kraepelin (17)). Bleuler (18) attempted to bring order to this confusing field of syndromes by applying the concepts of hereditary psychopathic disposition but his views did not gain ground in the English literature. Bowman (19) in 1936 followed Meyer in postulating that the different syndromes discussed under the heading of alcoholic psychoses do not constitute distinct disease categories, merely common and typical ways in which the individual suffering from excessive alcohol consumption over a prolonged time may react. On the other hand, French psychiatrists (20) maintained that alcoholic mental disorders should be classified and subdivided into numerous categories and subtypes, according to the findings on detailed clinical examination.

Bowman and Jellinek (21) in 1942 began to depart from the purely phenomenological classifications toward a system based on aetiological factors. They were enabled to do this by the discoveries of nutritional deficiencies in beri beri, pellagra, Wernicke's and Korsakoff's disease (22). Their work was completed by the Boston group of neurologists and neuropathologists, who established the most widely accepted system of aetiological classification of the effect of alcohol on the nervous system (23, 24, 25). The main categories of this schema are:

1. Acute intoxication: drunkenness, coma, excitement.
2. Abstinence syndrome: tremulousness, hallucinosis, seizures, delirium tremens, auditory hallucinosis.
3. Nutritional diseases: Wernicke-Korsakoff syndrome, polyneuropathy, retrobulbar neuropathy, pellagra, and probably cerebellar degeneration, central pontine myelinolysis, and Marchiafava-Bignami disease.
4. Neurological disorders consequent on hepatic disease: hepatic stupor and coma, and chronic hepato-cerebral degeneration.
5. Disease of uncertain pathogenesis: cerebral atrophy.

Tommasi (26) in France and Wieser (27) in Germany followed the above scheme, but attributed the cerebral atrophy to the chronic, direct toxic effect of alcohol and called attention to the possible role of head injury in the causation of some alcoholic brain disorders.

Courville (28) presented an alternative classification, based not on clinical features, nor on aetiology, but on the neuropathology seen in the brains of chronic alcoholics. He particularly emphasized the cortical atrophy of the frontal lobes, and claimed that alcohol was the most important cause of this degeneration in the presenium.

In the light of the availability of aetiological and pathological classifications, it is curious that the official system of the APA, the DSM II, (and the systems used in most textbooks of psychiatry) are still phrased in phenomenological terms. It is more disturbing that the DSM II appears to ignore some of the recent advances even in the field of clinical descriptions.

Another common way of classification is to divide the brain syndromes into acute, reversible and chronic, irreversible categories (29). That this distinction is not watertight was shown by Bennett (30) who described an intermediate phase of alcoholic brain disease.

In this paper only a passing mention can be made of the acute syndromes, so that the clinical features of chronic, intermediate and subclinical brain damage associated with alcoholism could be discussed.

REVIEW OF CLINICAL FEATURES

Korsakoff's Psychosis

The best documented description of the mental state of patients with this disorder comes from Victor, Adams and Collins (31) and from Talland (32). The two essential features of the condition appear to be: retrograde amnesia (inability to recall some events that occurred before the onset of the disease); and anterograde amnesia (impaired ability to form new memories). Korsakoff syndrome patients are otherwise alert, show no apraxia or other cortical signs, and their social behaviour is normal within the limits of their memory impairment. At times a mild perceptual and conceptual disorder, usually detectable only on psychological testing, accompanies the memory loss. While Talland regarded this as a part of the memory disorder, Adams (31) considered it a coincidental feature, seen only in alcoholic cases of the amnesic syndrome. His view is supported by a review of the literature. Korsakoff's original alcoholic patients demonstrated some cortical signs, while his non-alcoholic patients did not (11, 13). Bowman and Jellinek (1) recognized the central, severe memory impairment, but also noted descriptions of aphasia, agraphia and stereotypy of speech. Kraepelin (17) and Bonhoeffer (14, 16) noted signs and symptoms that are suggestive of cortical injury in addition to the memory defect. Recent review of the clinicopathological correlations of the amnesic syndrome established that the essential defect for the Korsakovian memory defect lies in the diencephalon (31, 33). Yet in some of the cases of Korsakoff's psychosis, cortical atrophy and cellular degeneration can also be found (31).

Confabulation, long regarded as a diagnostic sign of Korsakoff's psychosis, is not a universal feature of the syndrome, and it is seen more commonly in the early delirious or stuporous phase, than in the stable, chronic phase. It seems to arise from different psychic settings in the two phases as well. In the early phase, confabulation is the result of perceptual abnormalities. In the chronic phase, fragments of recent and remote memories are condensed and telescoped together, with disregard for temporal continuity.

While the amnesic defect is the distinctive mark of Korsakovian patients, and cortical signs may be found as coincidental features, the emotional state of these subjects is characteristically affected. In the early phase some fluctuation of the mood is common, but later a flat, detached state of apathy prevails. Affective changes are rapid and shallow, and the behaviour is distractable and inconstant.

The natural history of the condition is more variable than its symptomatology. The onset of the psychosis is marked by a global confusion, or a classical delirium, or rarely by a pure amnesic state. About half the patients show significant recovery, usually within the first three months, and the extent of recovery is not related to the initial severity of the disorder.

Dementia

Forms of dementia, with alteration of all mental functions, are not well described in the recent literature on alcoholism. The subject fails to rate a mention in Harrison's textbook of medicine and in Mayer-Gross, Roth and Slaters's textbook of psychiatry. Yet clinical experience suggests that the picture so well described by the early writers, and by some French authors more recently, still has validity. Hecaen and Ajuriaguerra (34) wrote: "as the intoxication progresses, one notes intellectual slowing and obtundation, imprecision of thoughts, a deficit of attention, difficulty with synthesis, troubles with judgment, . . . there is often euphoria, or passivity, but the mood can change to anger and the behavior can become aggressive." The clinical picture of some patients resembles that seen in general paresis.

The syndrome of global post-alcoholic dementia was associated with extensive cortical atrophy and ventricular dilatation in Courville's series of autopsies. The atrophy was more marked than that seen in cases of Korsakoff's psychosis. In the fifties, several papers (35-40) described the pneumoencephalographic appearance of cerebral atrophy in cases of alcoholic dementia. Neither the clinical assessment, nor the grading of the X-rays was standardized enough to permit a correlation between the severity of the dementia and the extent of the atrophy.

Alcoholic Deterioration

This term often appears to be used in an interchangeable manner with "early dementia". Bleuler (18) emphasized the ethical deterioration, impulsive brutality and labile affectivity of many chronic alcoholics. While orientation is normal in these cases, there is often an impairment of memory and deterioration of abstractive capacity and social judgment. The abnormality is more apparent on the level of conduct rather than in symbolic function.

Lereboullet and Pluvinage (41) noted that in many of their 88 cases of pneumoencephalographic cerebral atrophy, overt neurological signs were absent, and the patients presented a careless, euphoric appearance, showed poor judgment, and expressed ideas of persecution and jealousy. They emphasized the clinical resemblance of alcoholic deterioration to the frontal lobe syndrome, and explained it by the predominantly frontal nature of alcoholic cerebral atrophy.

Intermediate Stage of Alcoholic Brain Disease

Bennett's (30) description of this syndrome has certain similarities to the clinical picture of deterioration: emotional lability, sociopathic behaviour, frequent amnesic episodes or "blanks", exaggeration of preexisting personality disturbances. He added an important temporal dimension to the syndrome: after prolonged abstinence there is a gradual clinical improvement, often paralleled by the improvement in the electroencephalogram. A recent report by Smith and Layden (42) also showed a gradual recovery in reaction speed, abstract thinking and field dependence in alcoholics after six weeks of hospital treatment. It is important to note however, that even some apparently severe, chronic cases of dementia or Korsakoff's psychosis may be partly reversible, and the "intermediate stage" refers not only to slow recovery but also to intermediate severity.

Subclinical Organic Brain Disorder

This term implies that the relatively rough methods of neurological and psychiatric examinations fail to detect an abnormality that would point to an underlying brain disease. It does not mean that such brain damage may not affect behaviour in some subtle way, or that it may not interfere with the ability to perform well on some psychometric tests. While minor degrees of brain damage may be inferred from a detailed examination of behaviour, the only certain diagnosis results from the demonstration of actual tissue loss or replacement.

That subclinical damage exists was shown by Courville in his chapter on alcoholic atrophy of the cerebral cortex. He did not produce figures as to the frequency of such lesions in otherwise normal alcoholics. Neuburger (43) found that less than 50% of 42 alcoholic brains were atrophied. Cortical atrophy and ventricular dilatation was seen in 25% of 62 autopsied cases of the Wernicke-Korsakoff disease (31).

It is difficult to know the indications for pneumoencephalography in some of the brief published accounts of cortical atrophy seen in alcoholics. While Pluvinage (44), Barini and da Silva (45), Pozsgai (40) and Tumarkin (46) all found a high proportion of cerebral atrophy in non-psychotic alcoholics, their case descriptions do not exclude the possibility that minor degrees of brain damage were clinically noticeable in their patients.

Bratfos and Sagedal (47) carried out the first unselective neuro-psychiatric assessment in alcoholics, and found some atrophy in 17 of their 19 patients; only the two young subjects escaped it.

Haug (48) performed pneumoencephalograms on 60 consecutive admissions for alcoholism, and found that 44 of these had some abnormality. The duration of alcohol abuse and the quantity consumed were related to the severity of the atrophy. Atrophy was also more common (in fact universal) among the malnourished subjects, but half of the well-nourished subjects also showed brain damage. The clinical features of this group were unremarkable: only 21 of the 44 brain-damaged subjects manifested any personality deterioration suggestive of frontal lobe affliction, and none of the patients was demented.

Brewer and Perrett (49) carried out a well designed PEG, EEG, and psychometric study of 33 well-nourished heavy drinkers, all under 60. The PEG was abnormal in 70%, the WAIS and Benton Visual Retention tests in 58% of cases, and there was only one case of clinical organic brain syndrome. Cortical atrophy was more related to psychometric impairment than ventricular dilatation, while the latter was more related to the age of the subjects. The authors did not comment on the possible effects of this subclinical brain injury on the personality or the behaviour of their patients.

There is now an extensive literature on the neuropsychological indices of subclinical brain damage in alcoholics. Two factors emerged from a review (50) of the subject: the loss of the abstract attitude, and the impairment of complex perceptual-motor abilities. These effects are consistent with the thesis that the effect of chronic excessive ingestion of alcohol is to hasten and accentuate the ageing process of the brain.

SUBJECTS AND METHODS

In 1964, the Alcoholism Clinic was established jointly by the University of Melbourne Department of Medicine and St. Vincent's Hospital, Melbourne, as a therapeutic and research unit. The major area of investigation of this clinic is the natural history of alcoholism and its medical complications. Of the patients referred to the clinic between July, 1964 and August, 1969, 1100 were considered to be suffering from alcoholism, this diagnosis being based on evidence of physical, mental or social disorders occurring as a consequence of prolonged excessive consumption of alcohol.

One hundred alcoholic patients in this group were diagnosed as suffering from dementia (syn. chronic organic brain syndrome), based on evidence of chronic, progressive failure of memory, loss of intellectual function and personality deterioration. In assessing their mental state, attention was focused on conscious state, orientation, memory, content of general information, presence of confabulation and perseveration, ability to sustain mental activity, abstractive capacity, speech, constructive skills, presence of apraxia and agnosia, affect and mood, insight and social behaviour. Diagnosis, assessment and differential diagnosis of dementia from other cerebral disorders was accomplished by selectively supplementing clinical examinations with examination of the cerebrospinal fluid, skull X-ray, air encephalography, electro-encephalography, and psychometric testing.

To determine the factors associated with the development of dementia, a comparison was made between the age and sex distribution, drinking patterns, social circumstances and medical complications of the demented group and a control group of 220 consecutive patients referred to the clinic during its third year of operation. A later incomplete comparison of the demented group with the total population of 1,100 alcoholics has not significantly altered the comparative observations with the initial control group.

RESULTS

Sex

The demented group consisted of 65 men and 35 women, *i.e.* 6.6 and 21% of the male and female alcoholics respectively in the total sample of 1100 alcoholics.

Age at Presentation[1]

Figure 1 illustrates the age distributions of all alcoholic men in the total sample of 1,100 patients and men with dementia, and the male prevalence of dementia in the sample. On the horizontal axis is the age, grouped in decades, at presentation to the clinic and on the vertical axis the number of men. The total height of each column is equivalent to all men in that decade and the height of the hatched column the number of demented men.

[1]**Statistical method: Marshall's Group Data Test for comparing empirical distributions.**

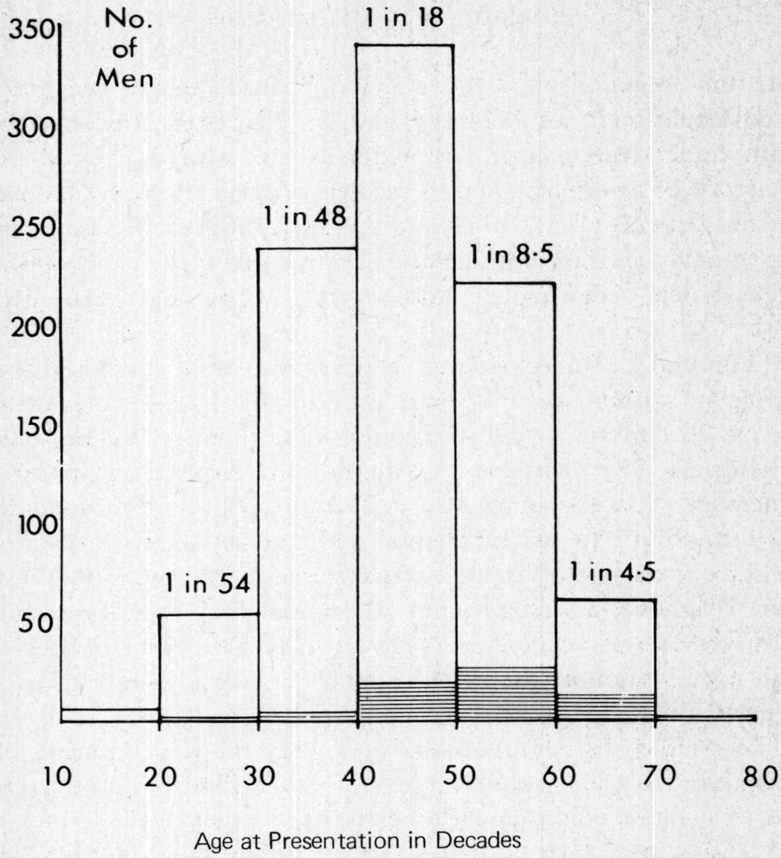

Figure 1: *Prevalence of Dementia in Alcoholic Men.*

The mean age of the demented women at presentation was 51 years (± 7) with a range of 37 to 61 years. The mean age of the control group of women was 47 years (± 7). The prevalence of dementia gradually rose from one in 28 in the third decade to one in 3.7 in the sixth and one in 3 in the seventh.

To summarize the comparative data on age and sex, dementia was approximately three times more common in alcoholic women than men and in both sexes there was an increased prevalence with age.

The demented men and women were significantly older than the control groups.

The mean age of the demented men on presentation to the clinic was 51 years (± 7) with a range from 24 to 68 years. The mean age of the control group of men was younger, 45 years (± 7), ($0.10 > p > 0.05$). The prevalence of dementia gradually rose from one in 54 alcoholic men in the third decade to one in 8.5 in the sixth and one in 4.5 in the seventh.

Figure 2 illustrates the age distribution of all alcoholic women in the total sample of 1,100 patients and women with dementia, and the prevalence of dementia in alcoholic women. The conventions are similar to those in Figure 1.

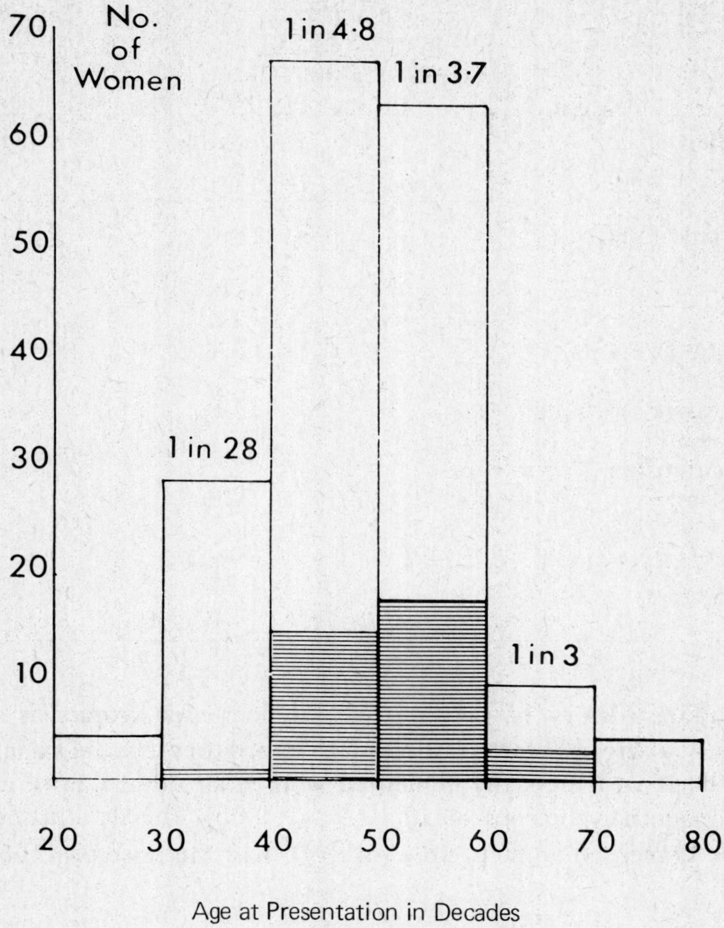

Figure 2: *Prevalence of Dementia in Alcoholic Women.*

Drinking History[2]

The drinking history of the control and demented men is summarized in Table I. The two groups started drinking at the same age. However, the demented men had been drinking both moderately and excessively (*i.e.* 100 gm alcohol per day) longer than the controls ($p > 0.001$, $p < 0.005$). The alcohol consumption was greater in the demented men, 300 gm/day, than the controls, 220 gm/day ($p < 0.001$) and the demented were more likely to be continuous drinkers.

[2]Statistical method: Marshall's stochastic analysis of empirically distributed data was used to determine the significance of the differences.

TABLE I

DRINKING HISTORY

Men	Controls %	Dements %
Age Commenced (Yrs.)	18.4	18.5
Age At Clinic	45.3	51.6
Years Moderate Drinking	7.4	11.7
Years of Excessive Drinking	15.8	20.8
Alcohol Consumption Grammes/Day	220	300
Pattern		
Continuous	77	96
Benders	20	2

The drinking history of the control and demented women is summarized in Table II. The two groups started drinking at approximately the same age. However, as with the demented men, the demented women also drank both moderately and excessively longer than the controls ($0.10 > p > 0.05$). The alcohol consumption was greater in the demented women, 180 gm/day, than the controls, 155 gm/day ($0.10 > p > 0.05$).

TABLE II

DRINKING HISTORY

Women	Controls %	Dements %
Age Commenced (Yrs.)	23.4	24.4
Age At Clinic	46.9	51.6
Years Moderate Drinking	10.1	11.8
Years of Excessive Drinking	11.7	15.8
Alcohol Consumption Grammes/Day	155	180
Pattern		
Continuous	88	86
Bender	8	6

To summarize the information on drinking, compared with the controls the dements, both men and women, had drunk both moderately and excessively longer, had higher levels of daily alcohol consumption, were more likely to be wine and spirits drinkers, and in the case of the men, were more likely to be continuous drinkers.

Social History

Occupation – Both demented and control groups showed a preponderance of "working class" patients, compared with the general Victorian population. However, no occupational group was over-represented amongst the demented compared with the controls. As might be expected, the demented had shown greater employment decline than the controls.

Education – The standard of education was similar in both demented and control groups, approximately 60% having received no more than a primary education.

Family integration – There was no difference between the marriage or the divorce rates of the dements and controls. The same percentage of dements and controls lived alone. The same percentage of men were living a "Skid Row" existence in the demented and control groups.

To summarize the social features, there was no apparent difference socially between the dements and controls for standard of education, "best" occupation and current degree of family integration. However, the dements had shown a greater decline in employment.

Clinical Features

Impairment of reasoning ability was present in all patients. Ninety-five percent had amnesia for recent events, 85% manifested abnormal behaviour and 81% showed abnormalities of mood – characteristically a steady apathy and often depression. However, 35% had emotional lability with swings from fatuous cheerfulness to paranoid aggression. Seventy-six percent were disorientated in time, 61% were disoriented in space, 56% had dyspraxia, 38% were confabulating, 33% were dysphasic, and 25% had perseveration. Most of the patients lacked insight, not only into their drinking problem, but also into their mental and emotional impoverishment. The severity of dementia varied from a failure of memory compensated for by rigid, obsessional orderliness, to a state of babbling incoherence and utter mental disintegration.

Distribution of the demented patients along a single axis of severity failed to disclose the heterogeneity apparent on clinical comparison. Several sub-groups were apparent. However, they did not represent watertight diagnostic groups but merely the way in which prominent clinical features clustered around each other.

Twelve were classified as "simple" dementia, the patients having poor reasoning ability and poor memory for recent events without any other outstanding signs. They frequently compensated for their defect by adopting a strict routine, and avoiding all threatening new situations. Their mood was characterized by depression and apathy. None of them suffered from Wernicke's encephalopathy, and malnutrition and neuropathy were less common in this group. Yet the daily alcohol consumption was higher in this group than in the others, and so was the incidence of delirium tremens.

Twenty patients displayed the characteristic absence of retentive memory seen in Korsakoff's psychosis. The onset of the psychosis was associated with Wernicke's encephalopathy in all cases, and all had some neuropathy. Other evidences of malnutrition were seen in 16 of them. Confabulation was a common feature of these patients, but it was not restricted to them. On the other hand, some cortical signs were detectable in most of these subjects, suggesting that at least in alcoholics in the first months of treatment, a mixed cortical-midbrain-diencephalic involvement is more common than the pure diencephalic amnesic syndrome.

Seven patients had impaired constructive, drawing or dressing skills and/or abnormal speech with mild to moderate degrees of nominal dysphasia, in addition to the disorientation, somewhat impaired recent memory and concrete thinking characteristic of the whole group.

Another group of 24 subjects displayed an outstanding lack of insight, motivation, and loss of internal control. Their behaviour showed little evidence of foresight and judgment, and was governed by the pressures of the environment. The behavioural anomaly was out of proportion to the modest impairment of intellectual capacity and memory.

Eleven patients showed some apraxia in addition to abnormal social behaviour, but still only a moderately impaired intellectual function. Twenty-two patients had a global, severe dementia. With their lack of verbal intelligence there was a lack of practical problem solving ability as well.

Air Encephalography

Air encephalograms were performed in 62 patients. They were not performed in patients who were too agitated to cooperate or who could not be admitted for complete investigations. The uniform findings were dilation of the ventricles, particularly the lateral ventricles, and widening of the cortical sulci. There was a low correlation between the degree of cerebral atrophy as demonstrated in encephalography and the severity of dementia. Atrophy of the cerebellum, particularly the upper vermis, was common; when present it was associated with persistent trunkal ataxia.

Differential Diagnosis

In addition to the 100 patients described with alcoholic dementia, a number of patients were found to have conditions which had to be differentiated from alcoholic dementia. These included anxiety neurosis, depression, chronic psychopathic personality, bromism, Wernicke's encephalopathy, subdural and extradural haematoma, cerebral syphilis and Huntington's chorea.

TABLE III

MEDICAL COMPLICATIONS

Complication	Controls (N=220) %	Dements (N=100) %
Periph. Neuritis	25	75
Wernicke's Enceph.	2	46
Malnutrition	30	51
Delirium Tremens	10	18
Epilepsy	10	18
Trauma	5	35
Cirrhosis	9	12

Medical Complications of Demented and Control Groups (Table III)

In the demented patients there was an increased incidence of other neurological complications of alcoholism. Peripheral neuropathy occurred in 75% of the demented patients in contrast to 25% in the control group. Wernicke's encephalopathy appeared in 46% of these patients. Fifty-one percent of the dements and 30% of the controls had clinical and/or laboratory evidence of malnutrition. While under observation, delirium tremens occurred in 18% of the demented group and 10% of the controls. Epilepsy occurred in 15% of the demented patients and 10% of the controls.

To summarize the neurological complications other than dementia: compared with the controls the demented group had an increased incidence of other neurological complications, some of which can occur as a consequence of vitamin deficiency alone, while others are still of undetermined and possibly multifactorial aetiology.

During the period of observation 35% of the demented patients suffered from trauma requiring medical attention and at times the injury led to more severe neurological defects due to subdural or extradural haemorrhage. Trauma occurred in 5% of the control group.

By contrast to the foregoing findings, it was found that there was no statistical difference in the frequency between demented and control groups of associated non-neurological illness such as cirrhosis, cardiomyopathy, peptic ulceration and chronic bronchitis.

Prognosis

The outcome in such an extensively cerebrally damaged group was as poor as expected. Only 14 patients showed significant improvement in their neurological and mental state. Only four of these improved enough to gain adequate motivation and insight to achieve voluntary abstinence. Forty patients required admission to long-stay institutions.

SUMMARY

Dementia, or chronic organic brain syndrome, is a relatively common complication of alcoholism, occurring in about 9% of cases. Its incidence rises with age, and it affects relatively more women than men. The condition has a poor prognosis for itself and for alcoholism.

Dementia is associated with a longer history of drinking and a heavier consumption of liquor than uncomplicated chronic alcoholism. Delirium tremens, general malnutrition, and specific deficiency disorders (Wernicke's encephalopathy, cerebellar degeneration, and peripheral neuropathy) are common antecedents of dementia. Head injuries are also common in the brain-damaged group, and may act both as causes and effects. There is, however, no excess of liver disease in the demented group.

Alcoholic dementia is not synonymous with Korsakoff's psychosis; the latter is just one of the syndromes within the wide context of chronic alcoholic brain disorders. Other syndromes include: frontal, parietal, fronto-parietal, and global disorders.

The clinical survey is presented in the setting of a discussion on the historical evolution of the concept, classification and current phenomenology of brain disorders associated with the chronic use of alcohol.

REFERENCES

1. Bowman KM and Jellinek EM: Alcoholic mental disorders. In Jellinek EM, ed., Effects of Alcohol on the Individual. New Haven, Yale Univ. Press. 1942
2. Wilkinson P, Kornaczewski A, Rankin JG et al: Physical disease in alcoholism: initial survey of 1000 patients. Med J Aust 1: 1217-1223, 1971
3. Huss M: Chronische Alcoholskrankheit, odes Alcoholismus chronicus. Stockholm, 1852
4. Sutton T: Delirium Tremens. London, 1813
5. Canton: Chronic alcoholism. Lancet 2: 237-238, 1860
6. Annan S: Idiocy from intemperance. Maryland Med Surg J 1: 333-334, 1840
7. Lawson R: On the symptomatology of alcoholic brain disorders. Brain 1: 182-194, 1879
8. Anstie FE: Alcoholism. In: Russel Reynolds J, A system of medicine. MacMillan and Co. 1868
9. Bevan Lewis W: A textbook of mental diseases. Charles Griffin and Co. 1889
10. Maudsley H: The pathology of mind. London, MacMillan, 1879
11. Korsakoff S: Eine Störung der psychischen Tatigkeit bei alkoholischer Lahmung. (author's abstract in) Arch Psychiat 21: 669-704, 1890
12. Victor M, and Yakovlev PI: S. S. Korsakoff's psychic disorder in conjunction with peripheral neuritis. Neurology 5: 394-406, 1955

13. Korsakoff S: Eine psychische Störung combiniert mit multipler Neuritis. Allg Z Psychiat 46: 475-485, 1890
14. Bonhoeffer. Der Korsakowsche Symptomencomplex in seinen Bezichingen zie den verschiedenen Krankheitsformen. Allg Z Psychiat 61: 744-52, 1904
15. Mott FW: The nervous system in chronic alcoholism. Brit Med J 2: 1403-1408, 1910
16. Bonhoeffer: Die Akuten Geistes krankheiten der Gewohnheitstrinker; Jena, 1901
17. Kraepelin E: Psychiatrie. 8th edn. (chapter: Der Alkoholismus) Leipzig, Barth, 1910
18. Bleuler E: Lehrbuch der Psychiatrie. (chapter: Die Vergiftungen) Berlin, Springer, 1937
19. Bowman KM: Psychoses due to drugs or other exogenous poisons. In: Blumer G. ed. The Practitioners' Library of Medicine and Surgery; Vol. IX., Sec. V., Chap. XIII
20. Voisin A: L'état mental dans l'alcoholisme aigu et chronique. Ann Médico-Psychol 3: 1-32, 1864
21. Leconte M, and Leconte-Lorsignol: Formes cliniques des troubles mentaux de l'alcoolisme. Arch Int Neurol 60: 218-221; 61: 12-23, 29-44; 1941-1942
22. Jolliffe N, Wortis H, and Stein MH: Alcoholic encephalopathies and nutrition. In: Jellinek EM, ed. Effects of Alcohol on the Individual. New Haven, Yale Univ. Press. 1942
23. Victor M, and Adams RD: The effect of alcohol on the nervous system. Res Publ Ass nerv ment Dis 32: 525-573, 1953
24. Victor M: Alcohol and nutritional diseases of the nervous system. J Amer Med Ass 167: 65-71, 1958
25. Adams RD, Victor M: Alcoholism. In: Harrison et al: Textbook of Internal Medicine, 4th ed. 1970
26. Tommasi M: Les encephalopathies des alcooliques. Rev. Lyon Méd 7: 215-225, 1958
27. Wieser S: Alkoholismus II: Psychiatrische und neurologische Komplikationen. Fortschr Neur Psychiat. 33: 349-409, 1965
28. Courville C: The Effects of Alcohol on the Nervous System of Man. Los Angeles, San Lucas Press, 1966
29. Thompson GN: Acute and chronic alcoholic conditions. In: Arieti S, ed: American Handbook of Psychiatry. New York, Basic Books, 1959
30. Bennett AE, Mowery GL, and Fort JT: Brain damage from chronic alcoholism; the diagnosis of intermediate stage of alcoholic brain disease. Amer J Psychiat 116: 705-711, 1960
31. Victor M, Adams RD, and Collins GH: The Wernicke-Korsakoff Syndrome. Philadelphia, F.A. Davis, 1971
32. Talland GA: Deranged Memory. Academic Press, New York, 1965
33. Zangwill OL: The amnesic syndrome. In: Whitty C.W.M., Zangwill OL, eds. Amnesia. Butterworth, 1966
34. Hécaen H and de Ajuriaguerra J: Les encephalopathies alcooliques subaigues et chroniques. Rev Neurol 94: 528-555, 1956
35. Maleci O and Fontanari D: Ricerche Pneumoencefalocisternografiche in casi di alcoholismo cronico. Atti Soc Med Chir Padova 27: 76-93, 1949
36. Peron N and Gayno M: Atrophie cerebrale des ethyliques. Rev Neurol 94: 621-624, 1956
37. Postel J and Cossa P: L'atrophie cerebrale des alcooliques chroniques, etude pneumocencephalographique. Rev Neurol 94: 604-606, 1956
38. Niedermeyer E and Prokop H: Zum klinischen Bild der Alkohol-Polyneuritis. Arch Psychiat Berlin 198: 274-286, 1959
39. Castro M: Alcoholic encephalomyelopathies — pneumoencephalographic studies in: Popham RE, ed. Alcohol and Alcoholism, Toronto, 1970
40. Tariska I, Gerèby G, Kardos GI: Tanulmányok az alkoholizmus pszihiátriai következményeiröl. Budapest. Alkohologia. 1971.
41. Lereboullet J, Pluvinage R, Amstutz A: Aspects cliniques et electroencephalographiques des atrophies cerebrales alcooliques. Rev Neurol 94: 674-682, 1956
42. Smith JW and Layden TA: Changes in psychological performance and blood chemistry in alcoholics during and after hospital treatment. Quart J Stud Alc 33: 379-394, 1972
43. Neubuerger KT: The changing neuropathological picture of chronic alcoholism. A.M.A. Arch Path 63: 1-6, 1957

44. Pluvinage R: Les atrophies cerebrales des alcooliques. Bull Soc Med Hôp Paris. 70: 524-526, 1954

45 Barini O and da Silva CP, Atrofias cerebrais em alcoolatras cronicos. Arch Neuropsig S Paulo. 17: 427-430, 1959

46. Tumarkin B, Wilson JD and Synder G: Cerebral atrophy due to alcoholism in young adults. U.S. Armed Forces M.J. 6: 67-74, 1955

47. Bratfos O and Sagedal E: (Alcoholism and organic brain changes) Nord Med 65: 139-143, 1961 (CAAL Abst. 9764)

48. Haug J: Pneumoencephalographic evidence of brain damage in chronic alcoholics. Acta Psych Scand (Suppl. 204) 135-43. 1968

49. Brewer C and Perrett L: Brain damage due to alcohol consumption: an airencephalographic, psychometric and electroencephalographic study. Brit J Addict 66: 170-182, 1971

50. Kleinknecht RA and Goldstein S: Neuropsychological deficits associated with alcoholism: a review and discussion. Quart J Stud Alco 33: 999-1020, 1972

The Nature and Significance of Neuropsychological Deficits Associated with Alcoholism

Elizabeth K. Warrington

INTRODUCTION

From a neurological standpoint it is helpful to categorize mental impairment according to level of breakdown. One convenient classification would differentiate impairments of attention, basic skills, reasoning or problem solving ability and memory. Attention, that is level of alertness, can be assessed using tasks of sound detection, threshold measurements or any task requiring sustained performance. Language functions as assessed by tests for dysphasia and visuo-spatial skills as assessed by tests of copying geometrical figures or the recognition of pictorial material are two examples of basic cognitive skills which are usually prerequisites to function adequately on more complex tasks requiring thought and reasoning. Reasoning and problem solving abilities are most directly assessed by the use of intelligence tests. Lastly, memory, the ability to retain and retrieve information from previous experience is perhaps the most elusive of mental functions to submit to quantitative measurement and analysis. All these facets of mental function have been investigated in the chronic alcoholic Korsakoff patient and impairments reported (1). Accepting that this is the case, it is important not to overlook the fact that there is very general agreement that a memory deficit is the cardinal feature of the alcoholic Korsakoff syndrome, the severity of which makes it most unlikely that this memory deficit is reducible to or can be accounted for by the more minor impairments in attention, basic skills and reasoning ability. I would suggest that these are associated or coincidental deficits. In this paper I shall discuss a small, selected group of chronic alcoholic Korsakoff patients who presented with a severe amnesic syndrome, other aspects of mental functions being relatively intact. A description of the syndrome and a brief analysis of the deficit is presented. (See also Warrington (2).)

SHORT TERM MEMORY IN AMNESIC PATIENTS

Experimental psychologists distinguish two memory systems – short term memory and long term memory. Short term memory is characterized by a limited capacity and short duration which has been estimated in the region of 20-30 seconds. That amnesic patients can have a normal short term memory is now fairly well established (3). The immediate memory span is normal in amnesic subjects for digits, sentences, spatial position of dots, etc. Moreover, on short term forgetting tasks they are not impaired. This has been noted using the Peterson technique in which a sub-span number of digits or letters are presented and recall required after a delay in which rehearsal is prevented by an intervening task. For delays of up to 60 seconds amnesics and normal subjects show the same forgetting curve. Amnesic subjects are not differentially affected by a distracting task over these short delays.

RETROGRADE AMNESIA

Retrograde amnesia (forgetting of events prior to the onset of illness) is a constant feature of the amnesic syndrome though estimates of its extent are very varied. Clearly there are methodological difficulties in assessing the duration of retrograde amnesia and heretofore much of the evidence has come from anecdote and unsystematic observation. Using questionnaires relating to public events in the past, we assessed memory for remote events in amnesic subjects. Compared with normal subjects amnesic patients were impaired for the whole time period sampled, 1930-1968. Similarly, on a test of recognition of well known personalities, contemporary figures and persons who had faded from public view at an earlier time period, the amnesic patients were consistently impaired even on the most remote experiences (4).

ANTEROGRADE AMNESIA

The anterograde memory defect is perhaps the most striking feature of the amnesic syndrome. Amnesic patients are unable to remember ongoing events. They fail to recognize people and places they are in daily contact with. The deficit affects both verbal and visual material; any retention task exceeding their immediate memory span is beyond their ability. Retention tested by recall and by recognition shows equal impairment (1).

INTERPRETATION OF THE AMNESIC SYNDROME

Memory mechanisms may be considered in terms of stages: input, storage and retrieval. Input of information into long term memory is considered to require a period of consolidation. One formulation of the amnesic syndrome has been in terms of a failure of consolidation processes. However, this theory has difficulty in accounting for the very long periods of retrograde amnesia described above. I wish to make the case for an alternative explanation. It has now been established that amnesic patients and normal subjects respond differently to different methods of testing retention. Amnesic subjects are especially aided by a 'prompting' or 'cueing' technique whereas this is not the case for normal subjects. For example, the amnesic patients' ability to recall or recognize words from a 10 word list was extremely poor, but given the first three letters of each word their performance was as good as normal subjects. Why then is cueing recall so beneficial to amnesic patients? One special property of this method of retrieval is that it eliminates incorrect false positive responses. That is, the patient is constrained by the cue and thus is enabled to reject any incorrect response not consistent with the cue. This finding clearly demonstrates that amnesics are able to store relevant information if the problem of retrieval is made easier. In other words, the information is in storage but there is difficulty in selection of the appropriate response (5).

These findings introduce the notion of an interference hypothesis. Can it then be shown that amnesic patients are more subject to interference effects? The cueing technique can be used to enhance interference rather than to eliminate it. In a series of experiments, subjects were tested on two successive word lists which had the property that the cue for an item in the first list was also the cue for an item in the second list. No impairment was demonstrated in the amnesic patients on first list learning but in certain conditions the amnesic patients were impaired on second list learning (6). That is, whether an amnesic patient demonstrates a retention deficit can be manipulated by prior experience. Clearly in everyday life, prior experience has the potential to 'interfere' with ongoing events.

CONCLUSION

The amnesic syndrome – a gross impairment of long term memory, in the absence of intellectual loss and with intact short term memory – is not unique to the chronic alcoholic Korsakoff psychosis. The amnesic syndrome can also occur following encephalitis and with bilateral hippocampal lesions. Though there are many differences in the neurological characteristics of these conditions, the amnesic syndrome itself is remarkably constant.

REFERENCES

1. Talland GA: Deranged Memory. London and New York, Academic Press, 1965
2. Warrington EK: Neurological disorders of memory. Br Med Bull 27, No. 3, 1971
3. Warrington EK and Weiskrantz L: The Physiological Basis of Memory. Edited by AJ Deutch. London and New York, Academic Press, 1973
4. Warrington EK and Sanders HI: The fate of old memories. Quart J Exper Psych 2, 432-442, 1971
5. Warrington EK and Weiskrantz L: The amnesic syndrome-consolidation or retrieval. Nature, 228: 628-630, 1970
6. Warrington EK and Weiskrantz L: The effect of prior learning on subsequent retention in amnesic patients. Neuropsychologia, 12: 419-428, 1974

Cerebral Disorders due to Drugs of Dependence and Hallucinogens

Myrddin Evans

INTRODUCTION

It is a matter of everyday experience that taking drugs of dependence in excessive doses produces directly or indirectly a wide range of cerebral injuries. Nevertheless we seem to have neglected to collect, sift and evaluate the mass of clinical data which is readily available to us.

The flat contradictions between the findings of different observers and the discrepancy in opinion expressed by equally experienced observers are highlighted in a brilliant review by Lewis (1), who deplores the dearth of experimental and statistical studies. Lewis believes there is justification for the outburst by Kalant (2) in her monograph on amphetamine dependence. She writes "These excerpts from the literature have been chosen to illustrate the degree of controversy that exists with respect to the addictive liabilities of the amphetamines. It is hoped that they also illustrate how the same evidence can lead to almost diametrically opposite judgments and conclusions when a scientific problem involves medical as well as ethical, social, cultural and other issues". There are in any case severe limitations on the interpretation of human data in relation to drug abuse; these include insufficient or inaccurate information (particularly about the dosage and identification of the 'drugs' taken); incalculable genetic and environmental influences and a multiplicity of potentially harmful conditions.

It seems that we are unlikely to make further progress rapidly without firmer evidence of cerebral damage and dysfunction than hitherto. Parallel experimental studies will be necessary to clarify issues raised by new clinical data because it is rarely possible to observe a satisfactory natural experiment.

The rapid advances in knowledge of the biochemistry of functional and experimental psychoses (3) and better understanding of the neuropathology of ageing (4, 5) provide new insights which will engender hypotheses applicable to drug dependence which can be tested by appropriate clinical studies.

It seems, therefore, timely to bring together the more recent clinical studies with the above attributes and refer to methods of investigation in closely related fields. Although tentative and speculative, it seems justifiable also to relate clinical phenomena tó biochemical aspects of drug dependence, affective disorders and psychoses. A more controversial and perhaps eventually a more important issue, is that of disturbance of personality; and whilst there is no satisfactory work to report, the possible physical basis of these changes must be mentioned. Attention must be directed to another important but neglected area, namely, the effect of drug abuse in the parents on brain development and cerebral functions in the foetus and newborn. The gross insults to the brain produced directly and indirectly by drug abuse are reviewed briefly in order to avoid repeated reference to the obvious, namely, that one such episode may leave residual deficits and disabilities which may alter the individual's reactions to various stresses including drugs. This must always be borne in mind in human studies of drug dependence, especially as severe assults on the brain are nearly always associated with coma or clouding of consciousness and anterograde amnesia.

These disparate, limited and rather subursine approaches to the cerebral disorders of drug dependence can be subsumed under four headings, namely, (i) severe brain injury, (ii) impairment of brain development, (iii) premature ageing of the brain, and (iv) functional psychoses.

SEVERE BRAIN INJURY

The grim catalogue of gross central nervous system terminal lesions occurring in chronic opiate and other addictions has been extensively reviewed by Roizin *et al.* (6). Findings include bacterial and phycomycotic meningitides and abscesses, subdural or cerebral haemorrhages, cerebral oedema and anoxia, and atrophy.

There is a dearth of studies that attempt to assess and record the tissue deficits which could reasonably be attributed to serious but non-fatal poisoning episodes. Neuropathological findings are in general non-specific indicating widespread damage and tissue death of a kind which occurs in any form of severe and prolonged hypoxia. Thus Weimann (7) found symmetrical softenings of the globus pallidus and early softening of the cerebral cortex including laminar necrosis of Ammon's horn similar to cerebral anoxia in cases that survived large doses of an opiate. Roizin points out that similar gross anoxic lesions are reported for barbiturates and cocaine, but apparently not for cannabis or the more commonly used hallucinogens. Cerebrovascular catastrophes attributable to amphetamines are well recorded (8, 9, 10).

Closed head injury is a frequent complication of the terminal illnesses of drug abusers. Brainstem lesions are common in patients surviving initial head injury in prolonged coma and must be kept in mind when interpreting postmortem changes (11).

In clinical cases there are the usual difficulties of unreliable information, multiple drug taking, the use of bizarre noxia, possible ingestion of metal contaminants and the unrecorded contribution to cell death of hypoglycaemia, hypothermia or hyperpyrexia. It seems incontrovertible that drug abuse can result in gross brain damage but it is obvious also that it is extremely difficult to disentangle cause and effect and seek for specific patterns in this extremity of pathology.

Careful study of the brain in patients who have stopped drug abuse and survived many years thereafter may show scars, atrophy and vascular lesions, but these are not uncommon findings in the middle aged and elderly (4). Findings in young patients would be easier to interpret given the rare conditions of adequate information, recovery from drug dependence and sudden death from some other cause.

The important questions are what are the long term effects of brain insults of a lesser degree but of the same kind? In man the accumulation of data of this nature will call for extensive record linkage and meticulous and painstaking neuropathological investigation in large numbers. More rapid and comprehensive studies could be carried out in animals, preferably primates.

A parallel with the slow if not slothful and tedious process of characterising the patterns of cerebral change which is the aftermath of boxing comes immediately to mind. The possibility that lasting cerebral damage might occur in boxers has been a controversial question since Martland introduced the term 'punch drunk' into the medical literature in 1928. The dispute continued intemperately until there were impressive neurological studies in 1965 (12) and 1969 (13) supported later by a number of neuropathological reports of a short series (14).

But as Corsellis writes (15):

> It is not easy to establish a pattern of damage or of degeneration in such limited material and most of the trenchant views that are expressed about the vulnerability, as well as the immunity, of the brain in boxing are still based more on supposition than on fact.

The appositeness of these remarks to the question whether lasting cerebral damage might occur in drug abusers is striking and one hopes salutary. Corsellis and his colleagues have in fact settled the question over boxing in their painstaking study of the brains of 15 retired boxers. They were able to identify a characteristic pattern of cerebral change which appears not only to be a result of the boxing but also to underlie many features of the punch drunk syndrome.

Amphetamines

The report of Citron *et al.* (16) which characterised a new disease entity attributed to drug abuse, namely, necrotizing angiitis (periarteritis nodosa) is of major importance. Prominent clinical features, evident in 9 of the 14 cases described, indicated in various degrees renal, gastrointestinal, pancreatic, cardiac or neurological involvement. The vascular changes including arterial aneurysms and sacculations were detected by angiography during life in the kidney, liver, pancreas and small bowel. The radiological changes were confirmed after death in three of four cases, no angiography having been done in the other. Widespread vascular disease was discovered involving medium-sized and small arteries in most organs and arterioles in the brain. They report:

> elastic arteries, capillaries and veins were spared. In acute lesions fibrinoid necrosis of the media and intima was prominent with a neutrophilia, eosinophilia, lymphocytic and histiocytic infiltration. Fresh occlusive thrombosis was common in early and later lesions. Subacute lesions were characterised by florid intimal proliferation with marked luminal narrowing. In some cases this lesion occurred in arteries with no other apparent damage, and in others, marked medial and adventitial alteration accompanied this proliferation, with delicate interweaving of medial musculature with new fibrous tissue. Older (healed) lesions demonstrated marked destruction of muscular and elastic components of the arterial walls, with replacement by collagen and a striking luminal narrowing.

Severe involvement of arterioles of the pons was found at postmortem in a 19-year-old man with a 2-year history of daily intravenous administration of methylamphetamine. Pathological findings in the brain are not specifically described in two of the cases, a 21-year-old woman who was a known heroin and alcohol addict, and a 47-year-old woman with a more vague history of drug abuse. Another 21-year-old woman with a 3-year history of intravenous use of methamphetamine, heroin, dextroamphetamine and barbiturates had 'destructive' arterial lesions in many viscera and tissues including cerebrum, cerebellum and brainstem.

Of the non-fatal patients, five had a history of methamphetamine abuse and showed typical lesions on renal angiography but did not have the usual clinical features. Methamphetamine seems to have been the common denominator having been used in large doses in eleven and exclusively in one. Apparently, in a separate study, four patients who had taken multiple drugs (but not methamphetamine) intravenously, and five patients who had used intravenous heroin and cocaine exclusively, did not show any evidence of the disease when examined clinically and by selective angiography.

Not unreasonably the authors conclude that drug abuse may be a factor in necrotizing angiitis. Methamphetamine may be a causative agent but other drugs and substances cannot be excluded. In the two case reports with specific references to lesions in the brain there is a striking poverty of localising neurological signs during life. One of these patients had a normal midline echoencephalogram and normal findings at lumbar puncture. Histological evidence of subacute and old healed vascular lesions is also of great interest as they suggest repeated episodes and the possibility of partial recovery. Hypertension was a clinical finding in the fatal cases but in only one other. The vascular lesions described are different from those usually attributable to hypertension.

IMPAIRED BRAIN DEVELOPMENT

Until very recently there has been a surprising lack of interest in the mutagenic and teratogenic potential in drugs of dependence (17, 18). Screening of the young population need not be a very sophisticated procedure. A fairly simple examination suffices to detect significant neurodevelopmental disorder as is shown in a study which found the condition in 6% of school-entrants in an English county (19). Over half of the children whose neurodevelopmental status indicated the likelihood of forthcoming difficulties were in trouble 3 or 4 years later. No doubt a more extensive examination would have picked up a larger number of minor abnormalities. However, the task of identifying the environmental contribution to this neurodevelopmental delay or defect is very difficult and expensive. But in view of the widespread use of drugs of dependence all over the world it is a matter which should be pursued vigorously.

There is now no doubt that a mother who smokes during pregnancy may by so doing retard the growth of her unborn child (20), but it is debatable whether this has a significant effect on brain development.

Analgesic drugs in high dosage are suspect. A retrospective enquiry of 833 pregnancies which resulted in the birth of infants with congenital malformations suggested that either salicylates or the conditions for which they were given had a teratogenic effect (21).

It has been shown in animals that drugs taken by the mother may not show deleterious effects in the progeny until a long time after birth. Thus in experimental studies in mice chlorpromazine and chloroquine have been shown (22) to cross the placenta readily and accumulate preferentially in the eyes of mothers and foetuses where they persisted for several months. If these observations in experimental animals reflect what happens in man there is a grave risk of retinal damage to the foetus when either chlorpromazine or chloroquine is given to pregnant women. Visual impairment and the appearance of retinal damage may be delayed until long after birth, however, and there is therefore a need for carefully controlled retrospective and prospective studies of children born to women who have been given the compounds (23). Whether such considerations apply for the drugs commonly abused is unknown.

Cannabis

Teratogenic effects have been reported in offspring of pregnant mothers chronically using cannabis (24). However the mothers in these two case reports also had LSD intoxications during the pregnancy. In their interesting study on pregnant mice Harbison and Mantilla-Plata (25) report for the first time two periods of gestational period susceptibility to Δ^9-THC, one period at days 8 and 9 of greater lethal action and another two days 10 and 11 which were the period of greater susceptibility to growth retardation. These periods of increased susceptibility have not been described in man. But if they exist the prolonged stay of a small proportion of a dose of cannabis in fat and elsewhere and the recycling of the cannabinols within the body would make it difficult for a chronic smoker to avoid risk.

Malnutrition

Malnutrition imposed at a critical period of brain development is likely to cause permanent impairment of structure and therefore perhaps of function (26). Dobbing (27) has emphasised there is a growth spurt of the human brain lasting from the last three months of pregnancy well into the second year. Hertzig *et al.* (28) showed that children who had been severely malnourished in infancy, some 5 years later were on average significantly inferior in their mental development to their sibs or to children in the same schools. The taking of high doses of drugs of dependence by the mother may have a toxic effect on nervous tissue in the foetus and interference with nutritional requirements of the growing brain. Despite the great difficulties and complexities in this field attempts must be made to answer the question whether drug effects on the foetus may permanently impair that individual's higher mental functions.

An impressive study by Jones *et al.* (29) strongly suggests that maternal alcoholism can cause aberrant foetal development in humans. Eight unrelated children of three different ethnic groups, all conceived by alcoholic women who drank excessively during the pregnancy, had a similar pattern of cranio-facial, limb, and cardiovascular defects with prenatal-onset growth deficiency and developmental delay. Undernourishment was not considered to be sufficient cause for the degree of prenatal growth deficiency found. Short palpebral fissures were present in all cases and this was interpreted as being secondary to deficient growth of the eyes. Prenatal growth deficiency was more profound in terms of linear growth than for weight growth thus contrasting with the findings when the mother is undernourished and the newborn is usually underweight for length. There was no catch-up in growth despite adequate nourishment and care after birth.

Of interest in the present context is the finding of impaired fine and gross motor function persisting in most of these children indicating some organic damage. In seven out of eight patients there was microcephaly which persisted from the neonatal period to early childhood. Five of the children were observed to engage in some type of repetitive self-stimulating behaviour such as head rolling, head banging, or rocking.

These findings, if confirmed, should lead to an intense examination of the offspring of all drug dependents and a search for periods of special vulnerability to certain drugs during foetal and neonatal growth. Efforts could then be directed to short periods of time during which the mother can probably be persuaded to reduce or cut out the drugs.

Other sources of neonatal and early retardation of cerebral development and personality include obstetrical difficulties of the pregnant addict (30), accidental poisoning, neonatal addiction (31), multiple drug use by children (32), folate deficiency (33) and harmful effects of withdrawal (34, 35).

PREMATURE AGEING OF THE BRAIN

Despite the remarkable ability of the brain to recover from injury (36), one of the most striking impressions in clinical practice with alcohol and drug dependents is the frequent occurrence of general dilapidation of the personality and loss of higher cerebral functions suggesting an accelerated ageing of the brain. This is particularly noticeable in young patients. But, regrettably, it takes a few years for this syndrome to impinge on the clinical mind, because at first the symptoms are interpreted as intoxication or as withdrawal states. Furthermore as we well know in older patients, diffuse cerebral destruction can present gradually and without localising signs or marked encephalographic or cerebrospinal fluid changes.

The review by Roizin *et al.* on the neuropathology of drugs of dependence provides ample support for the general statement that the drugs as commonly used can produce brain cell death, cell injury including accumulation of 'wear and tear' pigment and vascular lesions. It is not surprising to find numerous case reports attesting to loss of brain tissue at post mortem in drug abuse but there is a surprising lack of evidence of cerebral atrophy during life.

Mental Illness and the Ageing Brain

In a study of brain changes associated with age and clinical diagnosis in 300 consecutive postmortems in one mental hospital (4), neither alcoholism nor drug dependence was diagnosed. This otherwise excellent and painstaking work attests that even in this elderly population (mean age 70 years) cerebral atrophy was not found in a quarter of the patients; it was not infrequently absent into the eighties and a severe degree was seldom encountered even in the 'organic' group. The degree of cerebral atrophy increased within the group of organic conditions with the degree of dementia. Corsellis concluded that the ways in which 'organic' deterioration manifests itself during life are more often than not reflected in the ultimate appearance of the brain.

Alcohol

In a recent study (15) of the aftermath of boxing in 15 men it was noted that many of them had drunk heavily at some time during their lives but the cerebellar degeneration in the boxers was different from that seen in alcoholism (37) and the histological appearance of the hypothalamic floor was not that observed in long-standing Wernicke's encephalopathy.

Roizin *et al.* did not specifically mention the neuropathology of alcohol addiction but this is well documented and cerebral atrophy demonstrated by pneumoencephalography has been reported (38, 39, 40).

Nicotine

Nicotine may be of importance because of the use of fairly large amounts of tobacco to make a combustible mixture with cannabis resin. Tobacco retinoneuropathy, which sometimes progressed to optic atrophy, is now rare compared to the days when tobacco chewing was popular. Chronic nicotine intoxication does not seem to have been indicted as a possible cause of atrophy but it is believed to be an important factor in many vascular conditions (41, 42).

Amphetamines

Rumbaugh and his colleagues (43) describe abnormal cerebral angiographic findings in 19 drug abuse patients. The case histories were unreliable in many ways and more than one drug of dependence was used habitually. Furthermore, the methods and solvents used could have produced disease, and various bizarre constituents included urine, milk and mayonnaise. All these features made it difficult to attribute the changes discovered to any particular drug or combination of drugs. Cerebral arteriography showed a beaded irregular appearance of many of the cerebral arteries with irregular segmental changes of calibre and contour of the vessel walls. The most common finding was small artery occlusive disease indicated by short segments of slow flow and/or complete block. The clinical features included deep coma (2 patients), hemiplegia (four), subdural haematoma (two), epidural haematoma (one), seizures and head trauma (four).

The findings were quite marked in four patients aged 16, 18, 18 and 21 years, all of whom used many drugs. The authors make a tantalisingly brief reference to a number of cerebrovascular catastrophies attributable to amphetamines. Thus they excluded several patients with subarachnoid haemorrhage due to bleeding cerebral aneurysms in whom the bleeding occurred immediately following intravenous injection of methamphetamine, one patient with subarachnoid haemorrhage from an arteriovenous malformation in whom bleeding followed intravenous amphetamine use, and one patient who presented with an intracerebral haematoma in the basal ganglia and internal capsule following amphetamine abuse.

Perhaps it was these amphetamine catastrophies which made methamphetamine the drug of choice when they initiated their experimental studies with 5 adult Rhesus monkeys (44). 1.5 mg/Kg body weight of methamphetamine was injected on alternate days over a two week period. Two other animals received saline injections and all were subjected to a series of cerebral arteriograms and killed at fourteen days.

Despite some methodological shortcomings the findings are worth quoting in some detail. Of the five animals injected with methamphetamine and examined radiologically, three showed decreased calibre of some small branches of the middle cerebral artery and/or of the lenticulostriate arteries. Two animals showed marked general decrease of vessel calibre of small and large arteries. These changes were evident after one week of methamphetamine injections and there was further progression of the generalized spasm at the end of the second week in one animal. At autopsy the cerebral cortex and basal ganglia were soft, there were numerous petechial haemorrhages and blood was present in the subarachnoid space in these animals. Microscopy showed cerebral oedema and foci of ischaemia and infarction and widespread haemorrhagic lesions centred around arteriole and capillary segments. Most of these changes were present in all five of the amphetamine injected animals. The test animals had become hypertensive, slovenly and aggressive and in four of them injections had been followed by cardiac arrhythmias and a fluctuating cardiac output. The two control animals showed no radiological, clinical or pathological abnormalities.

Rumbaugh and his colleagues propose to make more refined studies with amphetamines and other drugs individually and in various combinations. Smaller dosages over a longer period of time might be useful in that they would not be as severe an assault on the brain. However, the findings in this experimental group provide a reasonable parallel to those in the clinical series and strongly suggest that widespread cerebral ischaemic damage may follow high dosage amphetamine injections in man.

Further studies of this type are very much to be welcomed. The experiments described give credence to case reports of cerebrovascular lesions due to amphetamines and will in due course clarify whether similar lesions can be due to other drugs, solvents, and injected particulate matter, particularly when accidentally put in an artery.

One of the important questions raised is whether there is a similar but less destructive process occurring at less extreme dosages. The variability of the clinical picture between individuals, and at different times in the same individual, is compatible with this, as is the frequent mention of clouding of consciousness, delirium, and delayed recovery. Many young addicts seek help after a particular episode of drug taking when they are frightened by features which are qualitatively different and leave residual defects in memory, concentration, and mood.

In ordinary cerebrovascular disease, similar episodes are rarely described in the early stages and may not be a feature in some cases of hypertension. In these conditions widespread focal damage can be found in the brain microscopically when there has been no clinical concomitant other than a general decline in energy and ability (4). There is a possibility that medium dosage amphetamine addicts may be prematurely ageing their brain due to widespread small foci of ischaemia. The clinical diagnosis of such a condition is unsatisfactory even with the aid of carotid angiography.

Stereotyped behaviour after large doses of amphetamines and phenmetrazine have been reported from several countries. Rylander (45) named this phenomenon 'punding' and described other dyskinesias including jerking of muscles and limbs, swerving and twisting movements of the body, fluttering movements of the arms and fingers, grimaces and champing of jaws, grinding of teeth and rolling of eyes, licking of lips, plucking of fingers and a variety of fixed postures and stereotyped gaits. These dyskinesias occur while the drug is still present in the body, but can continue for several days after its elimination.

In rats, stereotyped movements are dependent on the presence of dopamine in the mid-brain grey matter. Thus Randrup and co-workers (46) showed that the sterotyped motor activity in rats treated with amphetamine remains unaffected when the synthesis of norepinephrine from dopamine is inhibited. But when the synthesis of dopamine is also inhibited the stereotyped behaviour is prevented but can be restored by the injection of dopamine into the corpus striatum (47).

Analgesic Abuse

According to Boyd and Hottenroth (48) the prevalence of analgesic abuse in Canada is comparable to that of narcotic dependence. Addicted persons are generally female and over 40 and take from 25 to over 100 tablets of aspirin per day. The association between prolonged ingestion of analgesics containing aspirin and phenacetin, and psychiatric disorder and nephropathy is widely reported (49, 50, 51).

Murray *et al.* (52) found that 28 of their 65 patients persisted in analgesic abuse with consequent deterioration in renal function in 23 and death in 11.

In a further study (49) Murray delineated some of the differences between those who ceased abuse and those who persisted. The persisters had more often a previous history of psychiatric treatment, attempted suicide, abused other drugs, smoked cigarettes more frequently, were more likely to have intellectual impairment, and more likely to have suffered parental deprivation before the age of ten. There were other differences including a stronger psychic dependence and a larger intake of analgesics over longer periods. The persistent abusers had commenced their ingestion at an earlier age, usually late teens or early twenties. The Eysenck Personality Inventory scores showed that most of the patients were neurotic introverts and scores on the hypochondriacal scale of the Minnesota Multiphasic Personality Inventory suggested that those who persisted in abuse were more hypochondriacal than those who ceased. Murray concluded that analgesic nephropathy was psychosocial in origin in the geographical area studied.

Possibly a more interesting association emerges from his data, namely, the relationship between psychiatric disability including drug dependence, and intellectual deficit with an earlier age of starting analgesic abuse, a higher dosage of drugs and longer period of taking them. Psychological changes may have been produced by the chronic intoxication.

Greer *et al.* (53) described five patients, the oldest 67 and the youngest 31 years of age, who had taken excessive doses of salicylates over a considerable period of time. Agitation, confusion, memory loss, stupor, and coma were observed at different times during the course of the intoxication. Paranoid and hallucinatory behaviour was observed in two patients. Tremor or dyskinesia was observed in four out of five. Papilloedema was present in one patient and this subsided after a few days. Electroencephalograms were taken in two cases and these showed diffuse slowing.

Abnormalities of the EEG have been noted by others (54) in patients with analgesic abuse, and in a third of one series (52).

Whether chronic analgesic abuse can cause accelerated ageing of the brain is now a live issue as a result of another interesting study by Murray (55). Nine brains from patients with analgesic nephropathy were examined. Neurofibrillary change was observed in four and senile plaques in six of the seven phenacetin abusers. No abnormalities were detected in the two patients who had taken aspirin only. In all the phenacetin cases, senile plaques were present in the frontal, temporal and occipital regions, but they were always most obvious in the hippocampal gyrus. Granular vacuolar degeneration was identified in only one case.

Psychometric studies were carried out on eight other patients who had taken large amounts of analgesics but did not have severe renal damage. Four showed definite evidence of organic impairment, two a mild degree, and two showed no impairment. A further three cases were found who had clinical dementia in the absence of severe renal failure or other obvious cause.

The estimates of analgesic consumption in these patients ranged from 20 Kg to 110 Kg. The authors point out that no similar pathological changes were seen in two patients who had not taken phenacetin, nor in six other patients who died of chronic renal failure due to causes other than analgesic abuse. As phenacetin seemed to be the relevant drug, they introduce the interesting (and possibly very important) notion that prolonged abuse of this powerful oxidising agent may overwhelm the antioxidant protection of the brain leading to accelerated deposition of neuronal lipofuschin and the formation of neurofibrillary tangles and senile plaques. This possibility merits further investigation because it has important implications for the prevention of neuronal ageing and for treatment during the period of rehabilitation after cessation of the abuse.

Whiteford and Getty (56) consider that lipofuschin is the only consistent cytological alteration that can be correlated with the ageing process. This lipid residue which accumulates inside membrane-bounded particles is also called 'age-pigment' or 'wear and tear' pigment. The general development is described by Slater (57) as follows:

> lysosomes ingest lipid-rich material in relative excess. This slowly peroxidises and is partially degraded; the composite particle gradually loses acid-phosphotase activity and perhaps other lysosomal enzyme activities. The peroxidised lipid accumulates imparting the characteristic colour and substructure to the particle. An excessive number of lipofuschin-rich particles is an indication that a considerable amount of membrane engulfment has occurred.

Acetanilid is an oxidising agent closely related to phenacetin and was a compound used by Sulkin and Srivarnij (58) to test whether extrinsic factors influenced the senile pigmentation of nerve cells. Vitamine E, hypoxia, ACTH and acetanilid were shown to produce or increase the deposition of lipofuschin pigments in the cytoplasm of nerve cells in rats. It would be of interest to test phenacetin and other drugs of dependence in this way.

Cannabis Resin

A sample of cannabis resin is a crude mixture of cannabinoids, terpines, and occasionally alkaloids, the whole being of greatly varying potency. The mixture may contain datura, opium, or other psychoactive vegetable material, harmful contaminants, and be a 'rich compound of cannabis resin and human effluvia'. The cannabis plant is noteworthy for its plasticity and polymorphism (59). Lewis (1) has reviewed the medical literature and in relation to 'cannabis psychoses' writes:

> The Commissioners (Indian Hemp Commission in 1894) concluded, after an enquiry of still unequalled scope, that "the usual mode of differentiating between hemp drug insanity and ordinary mania was in the highest degree uncertain and therefore fallacious. . . The excessive use of hemp drugs may, especially in cases where there is any weakness or hereditary predisposition, induce insanity. It has been shown that the effect of hemp drugs in this respect has hitherto been greatly exaggerated, but that they do sometimes produce insanity seems beyond question. Nevertheless, it has been questioned. Even so guarded a statement implies that there are some sure criteria for establishing the causal role of the cannabis, either when it has been established that a man exhibiting a so-called "functional psychosis" had previously been for years smoking or eating cannabis, or when such a history precedes the onset of an "exogenous psychosis" exhibiting the cognitive and other defects attributable to physical or chemical damage to the brain. As a rule the writers on the subject do not

> give enough detail to warrant any attempt at retrospective diagnosis, but, in those who do, there are instances of persistent confusional syndromes shading off with the passage of time into chronic dementia in which the cannabis seems to have been the major cause.

This statement accords very well with the doubts, anxieties and clinical impressions which were the background to the study initiated by Campbell (60) following an epidemic of cannabis resin smoking and other drug abuse in the south west regions of the British Isles and Wales (61). This study was prompted by the finding of cerebral atrophy on air-encephalography in four young patients referred to Dr. Campbell for neurological investigation of headache, memory loss or behaviour change. A common factor in all four histories was prolonged heavy cannabis smoking. Since no recognised cause of the cerebral atrophy was apparent, neurological and radiological investigation of other cannabis smokers seemed indicated. The next five patients were asked to submit to an air-encephalogram to assess possible brain damage. All had a history of heavy smoking of cannabis resin and all agreed readily to the investigations suggested because they feared that they had sustained permanent ill effects due to drug abuse. Of these five, two were already known to me and the other three were the next cases referred to outpatients with histories of long-standing cannabis smoking. The last patient, making a total of ten men, was admitted with a drug overdose and had a 6-year history of drug abuse with heavy cannabis intake. We rejected several patients who had taken significant amounts of hard drugs, *i.e.* heroin, morphine and cocaine (62).

Because of the very nature of the test of air-encephalography we were limited in the population from which a comparative group could be collected to persons who had already had the test. The mean age of our patients was 22 years. The records of a complete series of cases referred to the neuroradiological unit for air encephalography in the age-group 15 – 25 were examined. The only cases excluded were those with abnormal neurological signs, a raised cerebrospinal fluid (C.S.F.) protein, or other abnormal features. None of the cases was excluded on the grounds of air studies alone and it should be explained that none of these cases had any condition likely to produce small ventricles. In fact, subsequent follow-up on all these patients did not reveal the development of any neurological illness or of drug abuse. In this way a comparative group of thirteen patients was obtained who if anything are weighted towards larger ventricles as they had been originally referred because of symptoms such as headache, loss of consciousness or syncope. Of the thirteen, seven were female and six male; however, the air-studies showed no sex difference.

The standard air-encephalography technique was used in all cases. About 25 ml of air was injected into the lumbar subarachnoid space with the patient in the sitting position under basal sedation. Just enough cerebrospinal fluid for routine laboratory testing was removed. Films of the patient's head were taken in this position, and again with the patient supine and prone. Routine views of the temporal horns were also taken. Measurements of the anterior ends of the lateral ventricles were taken from films obtained in the anteroposterior position with the patient supine. Measurements of the lateral ventricular size were carried out using three standard diameters, and an accurate area measurement was also obtained by using a planimeter.

The area measurement and two linear measures showed significant differences between the cannabis smokers and the controls and these results are summarised in Table I. There was no significant difference in the widest transverse diameter of the frontal horn, nor in the oblique diameter from the lateral angle to the junction of the floor of the body of the lateral ventricle with the medial wall. A line (column C) at right angles to the oblique, 5 mm from its lateral extremity, gives a measure of the lateral angle of the ventricle and this was more markedly different on the left ($p<0.001$) than on the right ($p<0.05$). The transverse diameter of the third ventricle (column D) was significantly different anteriorly ($p<0.01$) as well as posteriorly ($p<0.01$). The area of the shadow of the posterior part of the frontal horn of the lateral ventricle (column E) was significantly different from the controls on the right ($p<0.01$) as well as on the left ($p<0.01$).

TABLE I

MEASUREMENTS C AND D AND AREA MEASUREMENT E FOR THE CONTROL AND DRUG-ABUSE GROUPS

	C (mm)		D (mm)		E (cm^2)	
	R	L	A	P	R	L
Mean of controls	4.8	5.0	4.1	4.7	2.5	2.6
Mean of cases	6.5	7.6	6.0	6.7	3.4	3.9
P	<0.05	<0.001	<0.01	<0.01	<0.01	<0.01

C = distance across the lateral extremity of the lateral ventricle (see text)
D = transverse diameter of the third ventricle
E = area of the shadow of the posterior part of the frontal horn of the lateral ventricle.
R = Right L = Left A = Anterior P = Posterior
Analysis using Student's t test.

Besides these differences in the bodies and frontal horns of the lateral ventricles and in the diameters of the third ventricle there were other isolated abnormal features in the drug addicts. Temporal-horn dilatation was found in five of the cases, and in one of those the dilatation of the horn was the sole abnormality found. The trigonal region of the lateral ventricles as seen in the prone films were also considered abnormally 'square' in three of the cases, and surface air showed dilated sulci (>3mm) in two of the cases in the frontal region.

There were none of these abnormalities in the control group.

In summary, the films demonstrate a definite pattern of cerebral atrophy. Apart from the generalised dilatation of the body and posterior part of the frontal horns of the lateral ventricles, the most striking feature is perhaps, the dilatation of the lateral and to some extent the inferior angle of the ventricle, and the falling away of the floor, combined with the dilatation of the third ventricle. These appearances suggest that the worst damage is in the region of the caudate nuclei, basal ganglia and the structures adjacent to the third ventricle. The occurrence of an isolated temporal horn dilatation in one case is of interest, but in another four cases this appearance was combined with the generalised changes in the bodies and frontal horns.

Significant cerebral atrophy is rare in young people and none of the known causes was found in this series of ten drug addicts. We could not find any other constantly present factor other than cannabis smoking to explain our findings.

Our patients presented very similar clinical features to those described by Kolansky and Moore (63) in adolescent cannabis smokers. We were also much struck by the parallel between the picture shown by encephalitis lethargica and that of chronic abuse of cannabis and LSD. This was evident in some of our cases by a reversal of sleep rhythms, hallucinations and mental changes. It is worthwhile repeating our quotation from Hall's book about the epidemic of encephalitis lethargica (64). He wrote:

> If the public asylums have seen little of disease, the homes of sufferers and the police courts for juvenile offenders told a different story, whilst in adults the history of 'not being the man he was', inability to work, being irritable and difficult, a loss of memory and a falling-off in moral character are signs of this infection.

In encephalitis lethargica the worst damage was in the basal ganglia, midbrain, thalamus and floor of the third ventricle, and this is the area where we have demonstrated atrophy in our patients.

More recently we would perhaps be intrigued by a comparison with the psychological component of the 'punch drunk' syndrome in boxers. Corsellis *et al.* (15) quote Winterstein's impressions of about 50 boxers:

> Most of those badly affected showed an impairment of intelligence. A bad memory for recent events was very obvious. A characteristic sign of mental dullness is the ease with which these men have adjusted themselves to their fall from a comparatively brilliant position to that of poorly paid occasional labour in ordinary life. Some have great difficulty in concentrating and are garralous; others again may be paranoid and suspicious, others appear overcheerful. . .

Corsellis *et al.* describe pathological changes in the medial temporal grey matter, in the bodies of both fornices, mammillary bodies and septum in their forgetful boxers contrasted with four of the men who had no recorded disorder of memory. In them the degeneration in the temporal components of the limbic pathways was strikingly less marked or even absent.

A further report from Kolansky and Moore (65) strengthens their suggestion that some of their cannabis patients suffered actual brain damage rather than physiological disturbance. They present 13 detailed case histories of adults aged between 20 and 41. All had smoked cannabis fairly heavily over a long period. The clinical picture was of a rather stereotyped pattern of symptoms, which included headache, reversal of sleep rhythms, difficulties in recent memory, loss of interest in life goals and what the authors describe as 'mental and physical sluggishness'. That the symptoms began after the patients started the heavy cannabis use and then tended to fade out within 3 to 24 months of its cessation is put forward as prima facie evidence of a causal relationship.

FUNCTIONAL AND EXPERIMENTAL PSYCHOSES

Cerebral disorders due to drugs of dependence are often expressed in disorders of affect, sleep, consciousness and of integration and ego functioning. When severe, these disorders are usually contained within the terms, functional psychoses, affective disorders and schizophrenia. The commonly occurring psychotic symptoms can be discussed under two headings, namely, perceptual disorders and mood disorders. There cannot be much dispute that a sufficiently high dosage of drugs and hallucinogens commonly abused will give rise to functional psychoses in a varying proportion of human beings. It is necessary to bear in mind the caveats which should protect us from undue reliance on animal work and the provisional nature of modern theories on the biochemical basis of the functional psychoses. But with this done, it is very important to examine the links between these two broad groups of disorders. Man's folly and ignorance must not be allowed to mock the improvements made in the treatment of the naturally occurring psychoses by producing a new chronic mental hospital population of man-made mental disorders. In the following brief discussion of the subject I am deeply indebted to the writing of Weil-Malherbe and his colleagues (3, 66, 67, 68).

Perceptual Disorders

Perceptual disorders are the desired result of the hallucinogens. Some of the most dramatic effects of lysergic acid diethylamide (LSD) and similar drugs have been observed on the neural organizations in the brain stem and the thalamus usually referred to as the nonspecific 'reticular arousal systems'. Several groups of investigators have demonstrated that LSD, mescaline and the hallucinogenic tryptamine derivatives produce EEG desynchronization that is typically associated with alertness or arousal. Bradley and Elkes (69) suggest that LSD might produce this effect by acting on receptors either related to, or located in, the brain stem reticular activating system.

A second arousal system mainly involving limbic structures and the medial forebrain bundle has been proposed (70), and this limbic system appears to subserve arousal processes related to such basic processes as hunger, thirst, sex and emotional expression. There is experimental evidence in animals suggesting not only acute but long-term effect on this structure after a single dose of LSD (71).

Weil-Malherbe and Szara (3) suggest that some portion of the functionally significant serotonergic pathway from the midbrain raphe to various forebrain structures including the hippocampus (72) is selectively sensitive to LSD and to other hallucinogenic drugs and plays a particular role in the dual arousal system.

The decreased activity of some serotonin neurons in this system produced by LSD and similar compounds (72) could be a direct effect or mediated through inhibitory neural pathways from a closely related sensitive area (73).

In this manner a parsimonious hypothesis is suggested which satisfies two puzzling features of the effects of hallucinogens and related compounds namely (i) the remarkably small doses necessary to produce profound changes, and (ii) a physicochemical basis for the 'hallucinatory constants' *i.e.* the remarkably uniform phenomenology of perceptual disturbances no matter what the cause is.

If we now accept these two arousal systems, that is the reticular formation and the limbic system, as a working model, we can elaborate a little on its function. Routtenberg (70) thinks the reticular activating system is more important in maintaining the general arousal of the organism and providing the organization for responses, while the limbic system is more relevant to reinforcement mechanisms, the two being interconnected so that they can each suppress the other, thereby providing a dynamic balance regulating behaviour. Another view (74) is to allocate to the first system an arousal in response to external stimulation, while the limbic system subserves arousal processes related to internal drives. LSD and the hallucinogenic drugs in acting on the serotoninergic raphe system would disorganize the organism's integration of sensory information with the internal needs of the individual.

Weil-Malherbe and Szara take these ideas another imaginative step forward to complete the bridge between molecular and behavioural as well as between the animal and human reactions. They write:

> . . .it is tempting to speculate that the perceptual phenomena in man (decreased habituation to the novelty aspect of the environment, increased sensitivity to details, distortion of forms and shapes, synaesthesia, and sometimes hallucinations) would reflect primarily the malfunction of the first arousal system, while the emotional reactions (feeling of fulfilment, increased significance, free-floating certainty, euphoria, ecstasy, or anxiety, and so on) would reflect the abnormal function of the second arousal system. The more complex symptoms (regression, disturbance in abstract thinking, occasional paranoid reaction, and so on) would be the result of the disturbed integrating process in which both arousal systems take part and upon which the higher order psychological functions (that is, defence mechanisms, cognitive processes) are dependent in their operations.

These stimulating formulations combined with the notion (75) that disturbance of Kluver's 'hallucinatory constants' is the unitary explanation for the effects of all hallucinogenic drugs and that this is considered by Freedman (76) to be crucial in the individual and cultural use of these drugs, provide a useful conceptual framework for studies on the physico-chemical basis of drug abuse. Perhaps it is compelling to remember at this point that the physical damage reviewed previously in opiate poisoning, epidemic encephalitis, alcoholism, cannabis smoking, in the 'punch-drunk' boxer and in the 'punding' amphetamine addict involves parts of the brain wherein lie the crucial dual-arousal systems in man.

The link with alcohol is reinforced in the recent work on the biochemical aspects of alcohol addiction (77) in particular the suggestion (78, 79) that hallucinogenic tetrahydro-beta-carbolines may be produced by interaction of acetaldehyde (produced from ethanol) with biogenic amines.

The dual arousal system model discussed above has developed in parallel and contemporaneously with the concept that some schizophrenics and at least some psychotic depressives are functioning at a sustained high level of arousal (80, 81, 82). The similarity between psychotic states *as they occur in the community* due to hallucinogens, and subacute delirious schizophrenia is striking. Only a psychiatrist infected with hubris could claim to be able to distinguish between them on phenomenological grounds. The paranoid psychosis due to amphetamine poisoning can be indistinguishable from the real thing.

Mood Disorders

The association between abnormal moods and drug abuse is common; indeed a desire to elevate mood either to a state above normal or to raise the mood up to normal level is the avowed intention of many drug abusers.

Most, if not all, drugs of dependence tend to be preferentially concentrated in brain areas rich in neurohormones, and these areas are, of course, located alongside and below the ventricular systems at the base of the brain. When drug abuse has produced damage in these areas one should expect mood lability, inappropriate or inadequate mood responses or a chronic dulling of affective reactivity. This does seem to happen.

We have been particularly impressed by the frequency of affective disorders in chronic alcoholism and withdrawal. The inverse relation between liver tryptophan pyrrolase activity and brain 5-hydroxytryptamine (serotonin) in disorders of affect are well documented (83). Serotonin, as mentioned in the previous section, is also implicated in the action of hallucinogens and possibly in the mechanism of alcohol addiction. The synthesis of serotonin in the brain depends on the availability of circulating tryptophan which is largely removed by the liver through the kynurenine pathway. This pathway is governed by the first and rate-limiting enzyme tryptophan pyrrolase. Thus it follows that the activity of this enzyme is of prime interest in studies of alcohol and drug dependence and their associated mood disorders.

We found (84, 85) that chronic ethanol administration in the rat produces a sustained inhibition of the total liver tryptophan pyrrolase activity of about fifty-five per cent. Moreover, this appears to be due to complete inhibition of the apoenzyme activity by an NADH-mediated allosteric mechanism. This inhibition is reversed in these animals by cortisol administration and by withdrawal of the alcohol. Withdrawal after 10 and 20 days results in increases up to two and half fold above the normal levels of both holoenzyme and total pyrrolase activities.

Further studies (86) provide evidence suggesting that allopurinol inhibits the activity of rat liver tryptophan pyrrolase *in vitro* and after administration by preventing the conjugation of the apoenzyme with its haem activator.

The usefulness of L-tryptophan in the treatment of depressive illness is thought to be due to its conversion in the brain into serotonin, the metabolism of which is impaired in depression (83, 87). The inhibition of the pyrrolase activity by allopurinol (88, 86) suggests that the anti-depressant action of tryptophan may be enhanced by joint allopurinol administration. It may also have a place in reducing the chances of relapse in the critical months following alcohol withdrawal in man.

Chronic phenobarbitone administration inhibits the apotryptophan pyrrolase activity in homogenates of rat liver and subsequent withdrawal enhances the enzyme activity by 2.5 fold (89). The phenobarbitone inhibition may be mediated by NADPH which also acts by an allosteric mechanism. Perhaps other drugs of dependence inhibit the tryptophan pyrrolase when used over a long period and they may achieve this effect through a variety of mechanisms.

In addition to its role in mood changes we suggest (85) that the inhibition of pyrrolase activity by chronic ethanol consumption may be involved in the mechanism of alcohol dependence. As mentioned previously (77, 78, 79) current biochemical theories of alcohol dependence postulate that acetaldehyde inhibits the formation of biogenic amine acids and interacts with the intermediate aldehydes or with the amines to form addictive or hallucinogenic substances. Inhibition of the pyrrolase may divert more tryptophan towards brain serotonin synthesis. The removal of the latter by acetaldehyde could prevent the feedback inhibition of tryptophan hydroxylase by serotonin. More tryptophan can be converted to serotonin thus providing a favourable reaction mixture in which the concentrations of both biogenic amines and acetaldehyde are increased.

CONCLUSION

A wider reading of the literature than can be adumbrated in this contribution raises points of interest. Firstly there is the gradual evolution of the idea that drug dependence of any kind has a physical as well as a mental basis culminating in Paton's (90) useful working definition: that dependence arises when, as a result of giving a drug, forces – physiological, biochemical, social or environmental – are set up which predispose to continued drug use. Secondly, despite the variety of men, animals, drugs and conditions, one gains the impression that in fairly high dosage to the brain, (and this needs some time to achieve in some instances) the end results are remarkably similar.

The present contribution has been concerned with some of the more serious cerebral disorders. Mechanisms of injury seem to be vascular, anoxic or histotoxic. Very interestingly the target areas seem to be adjacent to the central cerebral ventricles. These areas might be especially vulnerable in the foetus and in the rapidly growing infant.

How this fits in with current theories about functional and experimental psychoses and with neuropathological findings in diverse conditions has been touched on briefly.

The temptation is to see a possibility of a sort of unitary theory at least for cerebral injury and for functional disorder in drug abusers. Perhaps the attempt should be made after deeper thought and study but it does seem very premature.

However it might be useful as well as provocative to theorise as follows: a serious degree of drug dependence and excessive use of hallucinogens produces functional and physical injuries in the reticular core and limbic systems, or put starkly – serious injury to the structures adjacent to the cerebral ventricles is an inevitable consequence of serious drug abuse.

One of the curious features needing comment is the occurrence here and there in the world, of a concentration of severe effects from a particular drug. This is useful in that it highlights the type of damage which may occur to a lesser degree generally, and this is well illustrated in the amphetamine cases described above. Probably some other factor is at work which intensifies the drug injury, perhaps this extra factor is genetic, viral or environmental. The latter category could include, for instance, subclinical lead poisoning or some reckless fashion of smoking cannabis which produces cerebral hypoxia. These possibilities should be borne in mind when investigating a new crop of serious cases and when carrying out experimental studies in animals.

It seems reasonable to conclude that (i) we should carry out much more intensive investigations on our ill drug abusers than has been the practice to date, (ii) in view of the vital areas at risk we should use the more sophisticated diagnostic tools more often; these include air-encephalograms and carotid angiograms, (iii) much more research is needed on every aspect of brain injury, including injury to the developing brain, (iv) the models of experimental psychoses such as suggested by Weil-Malherbe and Szara seem to be very relevant to the problem of brain injury in drug abusers and should provide a number of postulates testable by clinical observation, valid-nonexperimental and experimental studies in man, and lastly (v) for a little while longer it seems wise to hold on to the idea that the brain is the seat of the mind.

ACKNOWLEDGEMENTS

I wish to acknowledge very generous help and encouragement from my colleagues in Bristol, the late Dr. A. M. G. Campbell, and Dr. J. L. G. Thompson and Dr. M. J. Williams. Also from Mr. R. J. Dannatt, Librarian of the Welsh National School of Medicine, Dr. A. A.-B. Badawy, Senior Biochemist of the Addiction Unit Research Laboratory and from Mrs. M. Harrison our able and patient secretary.

REFERENCES

1. Lewis A Sir: Amphetamines, Barbiturates, LSD and Cannabis: their Use and Misuse. D.H.S.S. Reports on Public Health and Medical Subjects. No. 124. H.M.S.O. London 1970
2. Kalant OJ: The Amphetamines: Toxicity and Addiction (Brookside Monograph No. 5) Toronto, University of Toronto Press, 1966
3. Weil-Malherbe H and Szara SI: The Biochemistry of Functional and Experimental Psychoses. Springfield, Illinois, Charles C Thomas, 1971
4. Corsellis JAN: Mental Illness and the Ageing Brain. London, Oxford University Press, 1962
5. Wolstenholme GEW and O'Connor M: Alzheimer's Disease and Related Conditions. London, J & A Churchill, 1970
6. Roizin L, Halpern M, Baden MM et al: Neuropathology of Drugs of Dependence: Chemical and Biological Aspects of Drug Dependence. Edited by SJ Mule and M Brill, Cleveland, C.R.C. Press, 1972, pp 389-411
7. Weimann W: Gehirnveränderungen bei Akuter und Chronischer Morphium vergiftung. Ztschr. Neurol. Psychiat. 105: 704-751, 1926
8. Goodman SJ and Becker DP: Intracranial haemorrhage associated with amphetamine abuse. JAMA. 212: 412-480, 1970
9. Weiss SR, Raskind R, Morganstern NL et al: Intracerebral and subarachnoid haemorrhage following use of methamphetamine ('speed'). Int. Surg. 53: 123-127, 1970
10. Kane FJ Jr, Keeler MH, and Reifler CB: Neurological crises following methamphetamine, JAMA 210: 556-557, 1969
11. Crompton MR: Brainstem lesions due to closed head injury. Lancet i: 669-673, 1971
12. Spillane JD: Five boxers. Br Med J 2: 1205-1210, 1967

13. Roberts AH: Brain Damage in Boxers. A study of Prevalence of Traumatic Encephalopathy among Ex-professional Boxers. London, Pitman, 1969
14. Payne EE: Brains of boxers. Neurochirurgia 11: 173-188, 1968
15. Corsellis JAN, Bruton CJ and Freeman-Browne D: The aftermath of boxing. Psychological Medicine 3: 270-303, 1973
16. Citron BP, Halpern M and McCarron et al: Necrotizing angiitis associated with drug abuse. New Eng J Med 283: 1003-1011, 1970
17. Lloyd JP: Teratogenic effects of drugs. Proceedings of the Third International Conference on Alcoholism and Addictions, Cardiff Vol. 1. Edited by M Evans. Welsh Hospital Board, 1971, pp 199-201.
18. Beardmore JA: Mutagenic effects of drugs of dependence. Proceedings of the Third International Conference on Alcoholism and Addictions, Cardiff Vol. 1. Edited by M Evans, Welsh Hospital Board, 1971, pp 203-210
19. Bax M and Whitmore K: Neurodevelopmental screening in the school-entrant medical examination. Lancet ii: 368-370, 1973
20. The Royal College of Physicians, London: Smoking and Health Now, 1972, pp 95-96
21. Richards IDG, Congenital malformations and environmental influences in pregnancy. Brit J Prev Soc Med 23: 218-225, 1969
22. Ullberg S, Lindquist NG and Sjostrand SE: Accumulation of chorio-retinotoxic drugs in the foetal eye. Nature 225: 1257-1258, 1970
23. Lancet i: Drugs and the fetal eye (annotation), 122, 1971
24. Carakushansky G, New RF and Gardner LI: Lysergide and cannabis as possible teratogens in man. Lancet ii: 150-151, 1969
25. Harbison RD and Mantilla-Plata B: Prenatal toxicity, maternal distribution and placental transfer of tetrahydrocannabinol J Pharmacol Exp Ther 180: 446-453, 1972
26. Waterblow JC: Nutrition and the developing brain (Letter). Lancet i: 425-6, 1973
27. Dobbing J: (Letter) Lancet i: 48, 1973
28. Hertzig ME, Birch HG, Richardson SA and Tizard J: Intellectual levels of school children severely undernourished during the first two years of life. Paediatrics 49: 814-824, 1972
29. Jones KL, Smith DW, Ulleland CN and Streissguth A: Pattern of malformation in offspring of chronic alcoholic mothers. Lancet i: 1267-1271, 1973
30. Stern R: The pregnant addict. A study of 66 case histories 50-59. Am J Obstet Gynaecol 94: 253-257, 1966
31. Annunziato D: Neonatal addiction to methadone. Paediatrics 47: 787, 1971
32. Milman DH: Multiple drug usage by children. NY State J Med 72: 2793-6, 1972
33. Sullivan LW, Luhby AL and Streiff RR: Studies of the daily requirement for folic acid in infants and the etiology of folate deficiency in goat's milk megaloblastic anaemia. Am J Clin Nutr 18: 311, 1966
34. Tylden E: The effects of maternal drug abuse on the foetus and infant. Adverse Drug React Bull No. 38: 120-123, 1973
35. James DG, Walker AN, Turial J and Battesi JP: A tale of two cities: a comparison of sarcoidosis in London and Paris. Postgrad Med J 49: 86-89, 1973
36. Illis LS: Regeneration in the central nervous system. Lancet i: 1035-1037, 1973
37. Victor M, Adams RD and Mancall EL: A restricted form of cerebellar cortical degeneration occurring in alcoholic patients. Arch of Neurol 1: 579-688, 1959
38. Brewer C and Perrett L: Brain damage due to alcohol consumption: An air encephalographic, psychometric and electroencephalographic study. Brit J Addict 66: 170-182, 1971
39. Tumarkin B, Wilson JD and Snyder G: Cerebral atrophy due to alcoholism in young adults. U S Armed Forces Med J 6: 67-74, 1955
40. Kálmán P: *In* Tanulmanyok az Alkoholizmus Pszichiáthna i Követezméyeiröl. Budapest 1969, p 107
41. Juergens JL, Barker NW and Hines EA: Arteriosclerosis obliterans: Review of 520 cases in the special reference to pathogenic and prognostic factors. Circulation 21: 188-195, 1960
42. Wray R, De Palma RG and Hubary CH: Late occulsion of aortofemoral by-pass grafts: influence of cigarette smoking. Surgery 70: 969-973, 1971

43. Rumbaugh CL, Bergeron RT, Fang HCH and McCormick R: Cerebral angiographic changes in the drug abuse patient. Radiology 101: 335-344, 1971
44. Rumbaugh CL, Bergeron RT, Scanlan RL et al: Cerebral vascular changes secondary to amphetamine abuse in the experimental animal. Radiology 101: 345-351, 1971
45. Rylander G: Psychosis and the punding and choreiform syndromes in addiction to central stimulant drugs. Psychiat Neurol Neurochr (armt) 75: 203-213, 1972
46. Randrup A and Jonas W: Brain dopamine and the amphetamine-reserpine interaction. J Pharmacol 19: 483-484, 1967
47. Fog RL, Randrup A and Pakkenberg H: Aminergic mechanisms in corpus striatum and amphetamine-induced stereotyped behaviour. Psychopharmacologia (Berlin) 11: 179-193, 1967
48. Boyd EM and Hottenroth SMH: The toxicity of phenacetin at the range of the oral LD (50 days) in albino rats. Toxicol appl Pharmac 12: 80-93, 1968
49. Murray RM: Persistent analgesic abuse in analgesic nephropathy. Psychosom Res 16: 57-62, 1972
50. Gault MH Rudwal TC, Engles WD and Dossetor JB: Syndrome associated with abuse of analgesics. Ann Intern Med 68: 906-925, 1968
51. Murray RM, Timbury GC and Linton AL: Analgesic abuse in psychiatric patients. Lancet i: 1303-1305, 1970
52. Murray RM, Lawson DH and Linton AL: Analgesic nephropathy: The clinical syndrome and prognosis. Br Med J 1: 479-482, 1971
53. Greer HD, Ward HP and Kendall BC: Chronic salicylate intoxication in adults. J Am Med Ass 193: 555-558, 1965
54. Kasanen A and Valleala P: Electroencephalographic findings in chronic phenacetin abusers. Acta med Scand 173: 35-40, 1963
55. Murray RM, Greene JG and Adams JH: Analgesic abuse and dementia. Lancet ii: 242-245, 1971
56. Whiteford R and Getty R: Distribution of lipofuscin in the canine and porcine brain as related to aging. J Geront 21: 31-44, 1966
57. Slater TF Free radical mechanisms in tissue injury. London, Pion Ltd 1972, p 210
58. Sulkin NM and Srivanij P: The experimental production of senile pigments in the nerve cells of young rats. J Geront 15: 2-9, 1960
59. Schultes RE: Random thoughts and queries on the botany of cannabis: The Botany and Chemistry of Cannabis. Edited by CRB Joyce and SH Curry. London, J. & A. Churchill, 1970
60. Campbell AMG, Evans M, Thomson JLG and Williams MJ: Cerebral atrophy in young cannabis smokers. Lancet ii: 1219-1224, 1971
61. Warren Shan: Teenage Drug Dependence in Cardiff – A study of a small group of drug-takers. Proceedings of the Third International Conference on Alcoholism and Addictions, Cardiff. Edited by M Evans. Welsh Hospital Board. 1971, pp 85-105
62. Campbell AMG, Thomson JLG, Evans M and Williams MJ: Cerebral atrophy in young cannabis smokers. Lancet i 202-203, 1972
63. Kolansky H and Moore WT: Effects of marihuana on adolescents and young adults. JAMA 216: 486-492, 1971
64. Hall AJ: Epidemic Encephalitis. Bristol. 1924
65. Kolansky H and Moore WT: Toxic effects of chronic marihuana use. JAMA 222: 35-41, 1972
66. Strom-Olsen R and Weil-Malherbe H: Humoral changes in manic depressive psychosis with particular reference to the excretion of catecholamines in urine. J Ment Sci 104: 696-704, 1958
67. Bunney WE Jr, Davis JM, Weil-Malherbe H and Smith ERB: Biochemical changes in psychotic depression. Arch Gen Psychiat 16: 448-460, 1967
68. Weil-Malherbe H: The Biochemistry of the Functional Psychoses: Advances in Enzymology. Edited by FF Nord New York, Interscience, 1967, p. 479
69. Bradley PB, Elkes J: Effect of amphetamine and D-lysergic acid diethylamide (LSD-25) on the electrical activity of the brain of the conscious cat.J Physiol 120: 13 P, 1953
70. Routtenberg A: The two-arousal hypothesis: reticular formation and limbic system. Psychol Rev 75: 51-80, 1968

71. Adey WR, Porter R, Walder DO and Brown TS: Prolonged effects of LSD on E.E.G. records during discriminative performance in cat; evaluation by computer analysis. Electroenceph Clin Neurophysiol 18: 25-35, 1965

72. Aghajanian GK, Sheard MH and Foote WE: LSD and mescaline: Comparison of effects on single units in the midbrain raphe, Psychotomimetic Drugs. Edited by DH Efron, New York, Raven, 1970, pp 165-170

73. Koella WP: Discussion of insomnia and decrease of cerebral 5-hydroxytryptamine after destruction of the raphe system in the cat. Advances pharmacol b/B: 280-282, 1968

74. Grossman SP: A Textbook of Physiological Psychology. New York, John Wiley, 1967

75. Gomrich EH, quoted in The Biochemistry of Functional and Experimental Psychoses. Edited by H Weil-Malherbe and SI Szara. Springfield, Ill, Charles C. Thomas, 1971, p 329

76. Freedman DX: Perspectives on the use and abuse of psychedelic drugs: ethnopharmacologic search for psychoactive drugs. US Dept H.E.W. Public Health Service publ. No 1645. Edited by B Holmstedt and NS Kline. Washington DC. 1967, pp 77-102

77. Tabakoff B, Ungar F and Alivisatos SGA: Addiction to barbiturates and ethanol: Possible biochemical mechanisms, Alcohol Intoxication and Withdrawal Experimental Studies: Advances in experimental medicine and Biology. Vol 35. Edited by MM Gross, New York, Plenum Press, 1973, pp 45-55

78. Davis VE and Walsh MJ: Alcohol, amines, and alkaloids: A possible biochemical basis for alcohol addiction. Science 167: 1005-1007, 1970

79. McIsaac WM: Formation of 1-methyl-6-methoxy-1, 2, 3, 4-tetrahydro-2-carboline under physiological conditions. Biochim Biophys Acta 52: 607-9, 1961

80. Goldstein L, Murphree HB, Sugerman AA et al: Quantitative electroencephalographic analysis of naturally occurring schizophrenia and drug-induced psychotic states in human males. Clin Pharmacol Ther 4: 10-21, 1963

81. Venables PH and Wing JK: Levels of arousal and the subclassification of schizophrenia. Arch Gen Psychiat 7: 114-119, 1962

82. Kornetsky C and Mirsky AF: On certain psychopharmacological and physiological differences between schizophrenic and normal persons. Psychopharmacologia (Berlin) 8: 309-318, 1966

83. Curzon G: Tryptophan pyrrolase-A biochemical factor in depressive illness? Brit J Psychiat 115: 1367-1374, 1969

84. Badawy AA-B and Evans M: The effects of ethanol on the activity of rat liver tryptophan pyrrolase. Biochem Soc Trans 1: 193-195, 1973

85. Badawy AA-B and Evans M: Tryptophan pyrrolase in ethanol administration and withdrawal, Alcohol Intoxication and Withdrawal. Experimental Studies. Advances in Experimental Medicine and Biology, Vol 35. Edited by MM Gross, New York, Plenum Press, 1973, pp 105-121

86. Badawy AA-B and Evans M: The mechanism of inhibition of rat liver tryptophan pyrrolase activity by 4-hydroxypyrazole (3, 4-d) pyrimidine (Allopurinol). Biochem J 133: 585-591, 1973

87. Lapin IP and Oxenkrug GF: Intensification of the central serotoninergic processes as a possible determinant of the thymoleptic effect. Lancet i: 132-136, 1969

88. Curzon G: Effects of adrenal hormones and stress on brain serotonin. Amer J Clin Nutr 24: 830-834, 1971

89. Badawy AA-B and Evans M: The effects of chronic phenobarbitone administration and subsequent withdrawal on the activity of rat liver tryptophan pyrrolase and their resemblance to those by ethanol. Biochem J 138: 445-451, 1974

90. Paton WDM: Chairman's introduction, Scientific Basis of Drug Dependence. Edited by H Steinberg. London, J & A Churchill Ltd, 1969, p 3

Behavioural Aspects of Ageing

Jack Botwinick and Martha Storandt

Behavioural aspects of ageing are discussed here in a non-technical way in order that investigators, in as many research areas as possible, be apprised of some of the data and issues of concern to psychologists studying adult ageing. The relevance of this discussion for the present purposes rests on the assumption that both behavioural age patterns and behavioural alterations resulting from alcohol and drug usage stem from similar changes in central nervous system functioning.

An obvious note of warning is appropriate here: similarities and differences between age data and alcohol-drug data may not indicate what is superficially suggested. The comments of Harry Kay (1) and the late George Talland (2) may be cited to explain this. Both comments were made in the context of the controversy whether short-term memory (STM) and long-term memory (LTM) are subserved by the same or different mechanisms. Both comments are applicable to the relationship between age and alcohol-drug data.

Talland wrote that, if the slopes of the forgetting curves of STM and LTM are similar or even identical (if age patterns and alcohol-drug effects are similar), it does not follow that the mechanisms for both are similar – "these parallels. . .may be superficial and may reflect that there are only so many ways in which information can be forgotten or misremembered." (2, p. 96) (Age and alcohol-drug changes may reflect the fact that there are only so many ways in which change, typically deficit, can be expressed.)

In like fashion, apparent differences do not necessarily reflect different mechanisms. Kay wrote:

> To take a simple example, a penny dropped in water shows no observable effects apart from being wet, when pulled out at once, but if left in the

> water for a year the discoloration is obvious enough. Yet the chemical "mechanism" is not different. . .(1, p. 67)

With these warnings in mind, knowledge of ageing behaviour patterns may be very valuable to those investigators researching alcohol and drug effects. In the absence of further information, similar-appearing functions provide first level hypotheses regarding the possible mechanisms. If age patterns and alcohol-drug patterns are similar, inference and information as to mechanism in one domain can point to the direction of investigation in the other.

SENSATION

In studying the behaviour of old people, most psychologists find it more interesting to focus on broader aspects of function than the relatively narrow consideration of sensory function. However, so much of the daily life and needs of older people relate to, or derive from, simple sensory loss that it becomes important to focus on this problem.

Some of the best documented age-related changes are those pertaining to sensation. It has long been very well known that, typically, the old can't see well at close range; they have presbyopia (e.g., Duane, 3). It usually starts much earlier in life than many persons realize. Far vision, as, for example, the opposite end of the room, also declines with increasing age (4). Therefore, signs that the older person must read should be written in large print. The larger the print the better he will be able to see it.

Older people, compared to younger ones, typically need more illumination in the room to see well (5). Among the reasons which may account for this is that the size of the pupil of the eye decreases with age (6) allowing progressively less light to reach the retina. Again, this need for increased illumination begins relatively early in adult life. There is an approximate linear decrease in the amount of light reaching the retina from the 20s to age 60 years (7).

The lens of the eye tends to yellow with increasing age. The yellowing of the lens makes the color blue difficult for older people to differentiate. Differentiation among blue, green and violet is especially difficult for older persons; differentiation among the reds, yellows and oranges is easier (8). Thus, if color coding is to be used, colors at the blue end of the spectrum should be omitted.

Adaptation to the dark changes with age. Dark adaptation includes both how long it takes to see well in the dark and how good (at what level) the seeing ability is. It is clear that in the dark, older people do not see nearly as well as do younger people (9, 10), but there is controversy as to whether it takes older people longer than younger people to adapt to the dark. The Birren-Shock study suggested that the rate of dark adaptation was independent of age; the Domey *et al.* study suggested otherwise, *i.e.*, more time was needed by the elderly.

Hearing suffers in late life too. When hearing starts to deteriorate, the high frequency tones are the first to go (presbycusis). The tones at the lower end of the audible frequencies are easier for the elderly to hear (11). This becomes most noticeable at about age 50 with a tone of about 1,000 Hz. There is also loss across the board, *i.e.*, lower and middle frequency tones as well as higher ones. Thus, louder sounds are better for the old at all frequency ranges. Sometimes this makes for problems. Loud volume may be uncomfortable for others who do not have appreciable hearing losses.

Another problem in hearing is often experienced when many people are gathered in groups, such as at cocktail parties. It is difficult to carry on and hear the conversation because of the background noise – there is much masking of the signal. There is reason to believe that masking becomes a problem for the elderly. There may be far fewer conversations going on at one time, but the elderly may experience difficulty in sorting them out.

There are changes in most or all of the other senses too (12). Taste sensitivity seems to decline in old age (13). This has a tendency to make food unappealing. This sensory problem may be combined with other practical problems. How is the food presented? Is the person eating alone or with others? Food may be unappealing or unappetizing if the person eats alone all the time.

In old age, the sense of pain (14) and of touch (15) decline also. There is some indication that the older person may be less sensitive to heat or to sharp-pointed objects and, therefore, may not draw away from them as quickly. He may injure himself to a greater degree than a younger person would. The sense of balance sometimes becomes disturbed and can lead to falls and accidents.

PERCEPTION

The literature on perception is so diverse as to include responses to pure tones and to meaningful, complex stimulus arrays. An effort was made recently to integrate the diverse data, utilizing a model of "stimulus persistence" (16).

If two identical stimuli are presented in very close temporal order, the response to the second stimulus is different, at least it is slower, than it is to the first stimulus. It is as if the trace of the first stimulus persists, interfering with the processing of the trace of the second stimulus. An aspect of this theory or model is that stimulus traces persist longer in the nervous systems of old persons than of young ones. This is more a theory than a fact, but much data may be explained in this way.

Stimulus persistence theory explains well the fact that discrete, simple stimuli coming in rapid order fuse more readily for the old than for the young. This is seen for visual stimuli, *i.e.*, critical flicker stimuli (CFF) (17), auditory clicks (18), and shocks to the hand (19). Stimulus persistence theory requires extension or modification in explaining more complex perceptual processing. In integrating sequential information, stimulus persistence seems to interfere with perception when the stimuli are complex. However, when the stimuli are simple, stimulus persistence might actually help. For example, when the stimuli are complex, as in meaningful speech, they become less intelligible for elderly persons when the speech is rapid. It is as if the longer persistence of the auditory trace of one word or sound in a sentence interferes with the processing of the next word; with young persons this would happen at more rapid rates of speech. When the stimuli are simple, perception may be enhanced by the fusion based on the persisting trace. Unlike complex speech where fusion makes for confusion, simple inputs can be meaningfully additive, as a study on vision by Wallace (20) suggested.

Vigilance is important in perception. Studies show that vigilance behaviour declines with age; crucial in this decline is the rate of information change (21, 22). The faster the speed with which inputs follow one another, the greater the age decrement. In differentiating the 'signal' from the 'noise', the persistence of the trace of one of these (signal or noise) may be thought to interrupt the processing of the subsequent ones.

Stimulus persistence is but one theory or model found useful in integrating a wide array of diverse data. Another one has been elucidated mainly by McFarland (23); it takes the form of 'oxygen want.' Many similarities were noted by McFarland between ageing and anoxia, particularly in regard to sensory and perceptual performances. He indicated that many tests for high altitude effects, where there is less oxygen, give essentially the same results as do tests for ageing effects. Indentical causal mechanisms cannot be assumed, but striking similarities suggested to McFarland that impairment may reflect interference with the normal metabolic processes within the individual cells.

In perception, the afferent nerves conduct sensory messages of environmental stimulations to higher brain centres. These centres integrate the messages and relate them to what already is in memory. If the cells of the brain or lower centres are deprived of oxygen and thus do not function optimally, deficit performance would certainly be expected. Anoxia theory receives support in the hyperoxygenation work of Jacobs, Winter, Alvis and Small (24). Deteriorated elderly patients, breathing 100 percent oxygen under high atmosphere pressure, showed much improvement in performance.

TIMING AND SPEED OF RESPONSE

More time is needed in old age to carry out even simple functions. In crossing streets, for example, it is necessary for car traffic to diminish appreciably before crossing is safe. In supermarket or cafeteria type situations, choices are made and executed slowly.

There is a large body of research dealing with this slowing, and the research has resulted in a change of opinion regarding it. It used to be thought that the loss of speed associated with reaction and movement was due mostly to alterations in muscle and, perhaps, peripheral nerve systems. It is now thought that the alterations underlying the slow-down are more basic. It is thought that the central nervous system plays a role in this (15). Despite this, some aid to the elderly seems possible.

Even though only a small fraction of the total reaction time is taken up with motor function (25), and even a smaller fraction seems to be associated with the time taken for the stimulus to reach the cerebral cortex (26), and thus, most of the time is in central processing, it may be possible to manipulate conditions experimentally to speed up responses of older people.

Increasing the loudness of the auditory stimulus (27) or possibly the brightness of the light stimulus will quicken the reaction times of the elderly. This is not to say that the old will be as fast as the young, but performance of the elderly can be improved.

Old people can be helped to be quicker in responding in ways other than increasing the intensity of stimulation. When there is a change in the environment and this change comes as a surprise, the responder is thrown off guard and responds with relatively long delay. This seems to be especially so for the aged (28). Pitchers in baseball games and athletes in other sports make use of this fact of surprise by changing the speeds of their pitches and directions of their movements. When, however, there is attentive expectation of when and where the stimulus change occurs, when the place and timing of the stimulus are known, reaction time is quick. The older person can be helped in his slowness by arranging optimum stimulus and pacing conditions (29). This involves relatively constant or fixed conditions, and ample pre-warning or opportunities for preparation.

On high-speed turnpikes, for example, signs indicating approaching stoplights could be especially important for the elderly. Similarly, a greater time period in advance of a green light about to turn red may be desirable for the elderly. To some extent, the older driver arranges this by himself. He does this by driving more slowly. When elderly people are seen driving, it is not difficult to get the impression that many of them control the speed of their inputs by slowing the speeds of their behaviour. Whether or not this slowing is purposeful, however, is an area full of controversy.

INTELLIGENCE

The slowing in later life is so encompassing that it is seen in many aspects of function. It is seen in the measurement of IQ, for example. In the administration of the most widely used test of adult intelligence (WAIS), a bonus is given for quick response and no credit for some performances when latencies are too long. A controversy developed as to the meaningfulness of this type of IQ test for old people. This controversy was resolved to some extent when the WAIS was given both with and without time limits, and when the scores of the aged were found essentially the same in both conditions of testing (30). But, as with many of the controversies in psychology, the resolution is not complete. In the measurement of intelligence, the decision of which test to use, or what items to include in constructing a test is crucial. Intelligence is in part defined by these decisions, and age changes in intelligence are described by them. For example, a practical test of intelligence was developed with which subjects were tested on the use of the yellow pages of a telephone directory, on common legal terms, and on getting services needed in everyday life. A rise in scores through middle and later years was seen with this test, even when with conventional tests decline was observed (31).

Even though conventional test scores decline with age, this is not true for all functions. And, even when a test shows decline with one method of age comparison, it does not necessarily show it, or shows it to a lesser extent, with another. For example, it is maintained by many that cross-sectional age comparisons show decrement but longitudinal age comparisons do not. This may be a generalization too quickly accepted by many – too quickly accepted for reasons such as sampling problems (32). It is nevertheless true that the extent of differences among age groups in intellectual functioning is a function of the method used in measurement. More often than not, the following generalizations hold: IQ tests measuring achievement or stored information tend to show maintenance of function in later life. The initially more able remain more able, and may even improve some in this type of function. This is at least true in its broadest aspects. When fine distinctions and subtle nuances of verbal response are measured, advanced age may also be associated with decline (33). There is little question regarding manipulative skills, perceptual functions, and abilities of integrating new information. These decline, certainly as seen in cross-sectional studies. The greatest decrements are seen in the initially least able (34).

LEARNING

Since aspects of intellectual functioning decline in old age and since learning and intelligence go hand in hand, it may be expected that learning ability declines too. Does it? Much research has been directed to this question but with equivocal answers.

The most recent and better research has distinguished between learning as a process and performance as an act expressing this process. Often overlooked is the fact that what is commonly called 'learning' involves some behavioural expression which in itself is not learning. For example, we must speak or do something to demonstrate what has been learned. If there is disability in the effector process, in the speaking, then this may give the impression of a defect in the cognitive process when, in fact, this is not the case.

Most of the studies have been carried out with tests of rote learning of verbal materials. These point to an age deficit. But, when performance limitations are accounted for, learning is seen to hold up reasonably well; at least, the decline is diminished to an appreciable extent (35, 36, 37, 38). Among the performance limitations most often investigated is response slowing; fast stimulus pacing makes for poor learning performances on the part of the elderly. However, there are other kinds of non-cognitive limiting factors too. Memory drums, projector displays, and even research psychologists may be limiting in their strangeness to older subjects; they are very commonplace to young adults.

MEMORY

Memory and learning are difficult to differentiate. Learning is assessed by the memory of what had been recently experienced. Conversely, memory is assessed by what had been learned. Melton (39) pointed out that learning is conventionally measured in relation to a change from one trial (experience) to another, while memory is measured in terms of the temporal interval between the trials. In learning, the independent variable is the ordinal relationship between trials; in memory it is the time between trials, *i.e.,* seconds, minutes, days. The dependent variable, the change in behaviour, is often taken as an index of a change in a neural event or neural structure. This change is typically called an engram or a memory trace.

When tests of memory are made shortly after learning – that is, shortly after the 'registration' of information in the nervous system – the process has been called 'immediate' memory, short-term memory (STM) and other terms. When the time interval between registration and recall is long, the process has been called long-term memory (LTM). Whether STM and LTM are both served by the same mechanism is controversial, as has been indicated earlier. Two things seem indicated, however, in regard to the reports of studies on adult ageing. First, LTM is thought less impaired with age than is STM. Unfortunately, this observation is based more on clinical impression than on controlled study. For example, rarely, if ever, has effort been made to control for the meaningfulness or relevance of the old stored information. How well remembered is old information that is no more personally relevant than is the new information taught by the investigator? Even if this were known, it is extremely difficult to evaluate quantity of information such that it would be possible to say that more of the new is lost than of the old. How similar are the units or chunks of memory that are stored over a period of years to those newly acquired in the laboratory or clinic?

Second, memory loss in later life seems to be a direct function of age differences in registration, *i.e.*, acquisition. Once age groups are equated for acquisition, differences in STM are not prominent, or even apparent (40). This, plus the consideration of stimulus pacing speed discussed earlier under the heading, "Learning", cast uncertainty as to the scope and extent of memory decline in later life.

The assessment of memory decline also depends upon whether it is recall or recognition that is considered. Clearly, recall data suggest greater decline than do recognition data. In fact, Schonfield (41) did not observe any decline in recognition memory with age, although Erber (42) did. Recall, much more than recognition, is thought to involve "retrieval" of information in the 'memory store'.

PERSONALITY

When the stimulus, the environmental input, is simple and clear – as a loud pure tone, for example – there is relatively little room for personal interpretation of the stimulus. But when it is ambiguous or weak there is much room for interpretation: the nervous system processes complex information in individual ways based upon individual experiences; decisions and behaviour reflect this processing. Psychologists like to take advantage of this by using ambiguous and weak stimuli to provide a minimum of structure and thus maximize individual differences.

Ambiguous and weak stimuli make for uncertainty. With uncertainty there is an interesting error that old people tend to make. They simply fail to respond. They choose to do nothing that the experimenter calls a response. The young may guess, or may otherwise make effort to respond when unsure; the old tend not to do this. The omission error was interpreted in one study as "a defensive reluctance to venture responses for fear of recognizing their inadequacy" (43, p. 96).

The fear of failing often takes the form of cautious behaviour. While general cautiousness on the part of the elderly has been emphasized in several studies, it became evident in one of them that the cautiousness might be more in the nature of avoiding problems than in dealing with them timidly (44). The error of not responding may be part of a greater disengagement process, a process by which older people are thought to dissociate themselves from others and from activities (45).

Perhaps the least investigated area of ageing is the study of personality. Data from studies on personality are difficult to integrate; one reason for this is that many of the studies have used tests to describe traits or combinations of traits. So many different tests have been used that the trait list is long and sometimes conflicting.

Many of the investigators end their studies unimpressed by the scope and magnitude of changes with age in personality (46). Yet it is difficult to know what is impressive and what is not. For example, a typical finding with the MMPI is that there is a slight elevation of the D-scale score (47). There is a slight but consistent trend for greater depression among the elderly than the young. What does an elevation in the depression score, especially when slight, tell about life in the real world? Depression is seen clinically in old age, especially among the aged of poor health. The range of depression is from mild melancholy to severe affect states. Some experts consider depression as the cornerstone of ageing personality (48).

Hypochondriasis (49) and social introversion (50, 51) are also seen, but less persistently. Constriction is another characteristic which is seen. It seems to be prominent in the Rorschach protocols of older people. An example of what tends to be reported in Rorschach studies is: fewer responses, a decrease in the variety of content categories, and an increase in the responses based upon form (52). Individual differences are always stressed in these studies and, in fact, it is often reported that some elderly persons present just the reverse patterns. One series of studies showed that, when age comparisons are based upon intellectually intact elderly, the negative Rorschach indicators are not found at all (53).

The specific procedures, as well as the details of sampling, are important in describing age changes. For example, unlike some of the Rorschach studies, data based on a TAT type of test indicated that when constriction was seen it tended to be more with men under 65 than over. The area of personality study in later life seems to be an important one but much more needs to be done to provide a basis for meaningful generalization.

CONCLUSION

These, then, are some of the behavioural aspects of adult ageing. It should be kept in mind always that however great may be the differences among young adults in behavioural or physiological function, the differences among old adults are greater. This appears to be true in most all areas of function; it reflects the fact of different rates of ageing for different individuals, *i.e.*, different genetic programming plus unknown, random, environmental 'hits' in the course of living. This makes accurate prediction of late life abilities and status for any one individual very difficult, perhaps impossible. Most of what we have to say about behavioural aspects of ageing applies more to groups than to individual persons. It is like the actuarial tables of life insurance companies. People like to think that they can outlive and out-perform the expected averages, and they arrange – and should arrange – their lives in accord with this. But they had better not ignore the going odds or else catastrophe could be the consequence.

The betting odds indicate that difficulties arise in later life, not only because of decreased ability but because of alterations in the environment. As indicated, there is loss of sensory functions, of psychomotor speed, of memory, of other abilities. There is also loss of income and job; and, through death, there is loss of husband or wife and friends. There is a fast-changing world of increasingly altering values. Cultural or generational changes over time, rather than alterations in the central nervous system, may well be responsible for much of what here has been called age effects (54).

Similarities and differences between this literature on ageing and that of alcohol-drugs should be compared for what new directions and insights may be developed in both literatures. But the comparisons, as was indicated at the start of this review, must be made with caution and awareness of the potential pitfalls.

REFERENCES

1. Kay H: Learning and aging. Theory and Methods of Research on Aging. Edited by KW Schaie. Morgantown, West Va., West Virginia University, 1968, pp 61-82
2. Talland GA: Age and the span of immediate recall. Human Aging and Behavior. Edited by GA Talland. New York, Academic Press, 1968, pp 93-129
3. Duane A: Accommodation. Archives of Ophthal 5: 1-14, 1963
4. Chapanis A: Relationships between age, visual acuity and color vision. Human Biol 22: 1-33, 1950
5. Weston HC: On age and illumination in relation to visual performance. Transactions of the Illuminating Engineering Society, London, 14: 281-297, 1949
6. Birren JE, Casperson RC, and Botwinick J: Age changes in pupil size. J Gerontol 5: 216-221, 1950
7. Weale RA: On the eye. Behavior, Aging and the Nervous System. Edited by AT Welford and JE Birren, Springfield, Illinois, Charles C. Thomas, 1965, pp 307-325
8. Gilbert JG: Age changes in color matching. J Gerontol 12: 210-215, 1957
9. Birren JE, and Shock NW: Age changes in rate and level of visual dark adaptation. J Applied Physiol 2: 407-411, 1950
10. Domey RG, McFarland RA, and Chadwick E: Dark adaptation as a function of age and time: II. A derivation. J Gerontol 15: 267-279, 1960
11. Spoor A: Presbycusis values in relation to noise induced hearing loss. Internat Audiology 6: 48-57, 1967
12. Corso JF: Sensory processes and age effects in normal adults. J Gerontol 26: 90-105, 1971
13. Cooper RM, Bilash I, and Zubek JP: The effect of age on taste sensitivity. J Gerontol 14: 56-58, 1959
14. Schludermann E, and Zubek JP: Effect of age on pain sensitivity. Perceptual and Motor Skills 14: 295-301, 1962
15. Birren JE: The Psychology of Aging. Englewood Cliffs, N.J., Prentice-Hall, Inc., 1964
16. Botwinick J: Aging and Behavior. New York, Springer Publishing Co., 1973
17. Misiak H: Age and sex differences in critical flicker frequency. J Exper Psychol 37: 318-332, 1947
18. Weiss AD: Sensory Functions. Handbook of Aging and the Individual. Edited by JE Birren. Chicago, University of Chicago Press, 1959, pp 503-542
19. Axelrod S, Thompson LW, and Cohen LD: Effects of senescence on the temporal resolution of somesthetic stimuli presented to one hand or both. J Gerontol 23: 191-195, 1968
20. Wallace JG: Some studies of perception in relation to age. Brit J Psychol 47: 283-297, 1956
21. Talland GA: Visual signal detection as a function of age, input rate and signal frequency. J Psychol 63: 105-115, 1966
22. Thompson LW, Opton E Jr, and Cohen LD: Effects of age, presentation speed, and sensory modality on performance of a "vigilance" task. J Gerontol 18: 366-369, 1963

23. McFarland RA: The sensory and perceptual processes in aging. Theory and Methods of Research on Aging. Edited by KW Schaie. Morgantown, W. Va., West Virginia University, 1968, pp 9-52
24. Jacobs E, Winter PM, Alvis HJ et al.: Hyperoxygenation effect on cognitive functioning in the aged. N Engl J Med 281: 753-757, 1969
25. Botwinick J, and Thompson LW: Components of reaction time in relation to age and sex. J Genetic Psychol 108: 175-183, 1966
26. Davis R: The human operator as a single channel information system. Quart J Exper Psychol 9: 119-129, 1957
27. Botwinick J: Sensory-perceptual factors in reaction time in relation to age. J Genetic Psychol 121: 173-177, 1972
28. Botwinick J, Brinley JF, and Birren JE: Set in relation to age. J Gerontol 12: 300-305, 1957
29. Botwinick J and Brinley JF: Aspects of RT set during brief intervals in relation to age and sex. J Gerontol 17: 295-301, 1962
30. Doppelt JE, and Wallace WL: Standardization of the Wechsler Adult Intelligence Scale for older persons. J Abnormal and Soc Psychol 51: 312-330, 1955
31. Demming JA, and Pressey SL: Tests "indigenous" to the adult and older years. J Consulting Psychol 2: 144-148, 1957
32. Riegel KF, Riegel RM, and Meyer G: A study of the dropout rates in longitudinal research on aging and the prediction of death. J Personality and Soc Psychol 5: 342-348, 1967
33. Botwinick J, and Storandt M: Vocabulary ability in later life. J Genetic Psychol, 125: 303-308, 1974
34. Foulds GA, and Raven JC: Normal changes in the mental abilities of adults as age advances. J Ment Sci 94: 133-142, 1948
35. Arenberg D: Anticipation interval and age differences in verbal learning. J Abnormal Psychol 70: 419-425, 1965
36. Canestrari RE, Jr: Paced and self-paced learning in young and elderly adults. J Gerontol 18: 165-168, 1963
37. Eisdorfer C, Axelrod S, and Wilkie F: Stimulus exposure time as a factor in serial learning in an aged sample. J Abnormal Soc Psychol 67: 594-600, 1963
38. Monge RH, and Hultsch D: Paired-associate learning as a function of adult age and the length of the anticipation and inspection intervals. J Gerontol 26: 157-162, 1971
39. Melton AW: Implications of short-term memory for a general theory of memory. J Verbal Learning and Verbal Behavior 2: 1-21, 1963
40. Hulicka IM, and Weiss RL: Age differences in retention as a function of learning. J Consulting Psychol 29: 125-129, 1965
41. Schonfield D: Memory changes with age. Nature 28: 918, 1965
42. Erber J: Age differences in recognition memory. J Gerontol, 29: 177-181, 1974
43. Basowitz H, and Korchin SJ: Age differences in the perception of closure. J Abnormal and Soc Psychol 54: 93-97, 1957
44. Botwinick J: Disinclination to venture response versus cautiousness in responding: age differences. J Genetic Psychol 115: 55-62, 1969
45. Cumming E, and Henry W: Growing Old: The Process of Disengagement. New York, Basic Books, 1961
46. Neugarten BL, Crotty WF, and Tobin SS: Personality in Middle and Late Life. New York, Atherton Press, 1964
47. Swenson WM: Structured personality testing in the aged: an MMPI study of theorontic population. J Clin Psychol 17: 302-304, 1961
48. Zinberg NE, and Kaufman I: Cultural and personality factors associated with aging: An introduction. Normal Psychology of the Aging Process. Edited by N Zinberg and I Kaufman. New York, International Universities Press, Inc., 1963, pp 17-71
49. Busse EW, and Pfeiffer E: Functional psychiatric disorders in old age. Behavior Adaptation in Late Life. Edited by EW Busse and E Pfeiffer. Boston, Little, Brown & Co., 1969 pp 183-235
50. Gutman GM: A note on the MPI: Age and sex differences in extroversion and neuroticism in a Canadian sample. Brit J Social and Clinical Psychol 5: 128-129, 1966

51. Heron A, and Chown SM: Age and Function. London, Churchill, 1967
52. Ames LB: Age changes in the Rorschach responses of a group of elderly individuals. J Genetic Psychol 97: 257-258, 1960
53. Eisdorfer C: Rorschach performance and intellectual functioning in the aged. J Gerontol 18: 358-363, 1963
54. Schaie KW: Age changes and age differences. Gerontologist 7: 128-132, 1967

Chronic Effects of Alcohol and Other Psychoactive Drugs on Intellect, Learning and Memory

Donald W. Goodwin and Shirley Y. Hill

> In discussing the effects of alcohol on mental activity, it is important to distinguish between the transient changes in psychological functions following the ingestion of restricted amounts of alcohol and those ascribed to its continued use.

David Wechsler thus raised the issue of acute versus chronic effects of alcohol at a symposium in 1940 (1). He observed that studies of acute intoxication were superior to those of chronic effects because they could be conducted under controlled conditions. He concluded that acute and chronic studies were "mutually supportive, but whether they are interchangeable is open to question" – a classic example of fence-straddling much emulated in the literature to follow on the subject.

The problem of separating temporary from permanent impairment also exists with regard to drugs. Generalizations are made and warnings issued about the continued use of psychotropic drugs, but almost all are based on investigations of acute states, or uncontrolled clinical observations. As Wechsler noted about alcoholics, it is only when we study terminal cases that we "again find experimental data." And with regard to alcoholics, most of these data are derived from studies of a diagnostically restricted and relatively small group – those with Korsakoff's psychosis.

This paper will review studies which bear on possible, irreversible effects on intellectual functioning from alcohol and other psychotropic drugs, together with a discussion of methodological problems involved in studying chronic effects of drugs in humans. Those conditions almost certainly of nutritional origin, e.g., Korsakoff's syndrome, will not be discussed. Observations about clinicopathological correlations will be left for other authors, as will effects of alcohol and other drugs on sensory and motor processes. Suffice to say that, in the absence of demonstrable neurological impairment (usually of nutritional origin), there is little evidence that chronic use of alcohol permanently impairs sensory or motor processes.

ALCOHOL STUDIES

Intelligence Tests

In 1940, Wechsler administered his Bellevue Adult Intelligence Scale to 29 hospitalized alcoholics and reported they had normal IQ's (1). There was no decline of IQ with age, or evidence of gross intellectual impairment. Since then many investigators have tested the intelligence quotient of alcoholics and almost invariably report them as normal. In a recent study (2) of Vietnam veterans (average age 21), alcoholics in the group had a somewhat higher IQ then did nonalcoholics, a finding reported at least four times in the literature (3-6). The differences in IQ between alcoholics and nonalcoholics, however, are usually small and often can be attributed to sampling bias. Even in advanced cases of alcoholism, the evidence indicates that, in the absence of a gross organic brain syndrome, full scale IQ scores are not affected by long-term use of alcohol.

The tests generally used to test IQ are the Wechsler-Bellevue, Form 1, and the Wechsler Adult Intelligence Scale (WAIS). Both tests have subscales lending themselves to analyses of selective disturbances in intellectual functioning. They permit, for example, separation of verbal IQ from performance IQ. Wechsler, in his original study, noted that his alcoholic subjects did less well on performance than on verbal tests (1). In this way, they resembled persons older than their chronological age, since older persons generally do less well on performance than on verbal tests. As early as 1940, therefore, Wechsler introduced the idea that alcohol may cause premature aging, a hypothesis still in vogue.

Two subsequent studies (7, 8) reported that alcoholics did less well on performance than on verbal tests, but the implication that this constitutes evidence of alcoholic deterioration has been challenged by other researchers (9) who argue that splits in verbal-performance test scores indicate acute lesions, not chronic and diffuse ones, as presumably would be expected in alcoholics. Kleinknecht and Goldstein (10) suggest that perhaps alcoholics do less well on performance tests than on verbal tests because of alcoholic peripheral neuropathy. It is difficult to evaluate this possibility, since the physical health of subjects is rarely mentioned.

Subscales of intelligence tests have also been used to construct profiles presumed to be characteristic of alcoholism. In their excellent review of these studies, Kleinknecht and Goldstein conclude that no consistent subscale pattern had emerged from the dozen or so studies of alcoholics. Wechsler, for example, in his 1958 book states categorically that the alcoholics do well on the Information and Comprehension subscales and poorly on Digit Span and/or Arithmetic and Similarities. With regard to performance, they did well on Picture Completion and poorly on Digit Symbol and Object Assembly. When this pattern occurs in young patients, Wechsler said, it clearly indicates brain damage, often long before it is clinically manifest.

However, there has been little subsequent evidence to justify this conclusion. On only two subscales are alcoholics' performances consistent: Information and Vocabulary invariably are unimpaired. In four of eight studies, Object Assembly was impaired, and Digit Symbol was impaired in six of nine studies (10). As Kleinknecht and Goldstein noted, reports of no impairment decisively outnumbered reports of impairment (10). Most investigators today conclude that no single subscale pattern is characteristic of alcoholics.

Organicity Tests

Some authors (11, 12) report that certain WAIS subtests appear especially affected by brain injury, in particular the Digit Span and Digit Symbol subtests, but others challenge this point of view. Wittenborn, for example, believed analysis of WAIS subtests was of no greater value "as a psychometric supplement to diagnosis than an inspection of subtests for a few conspicuous instances of failure and relative success" (13). Given this uncertainty about the usefulness of general intelligence tests in identifying brain damage, the trend recently has been to apply tests specifically designed to assess organicity. These tests, as applied to alcoholics, will be reviewed.

Halstead Battery

Four groups have administered the Halstead Battery to alcoholics and compared the results with those obtained from healthy and brain-damaged subjects. The results have been remarkably consistent.

Fitzhugh *et al.* found that hospitalized alcoholics generally performed the tasks as well as healthy controls, with the exception of one measure of abstraction ability, the Category Test (9, 14). The Category Test utilizes a projection apparatus for presentation of stimulus material. The subject is required to "abstract" principles based upon variables such as size, shape, number, position, brightness and color and respond to one of 4 correct alternatives by pulling a lever. A bell is heard when the subject makes a correct response and a buzzer informs him of an incorrect one. The score is the number of incorrect responses. Thus, the test measures the ability to solve unique problems rather than those dependent upon possession of prior information.

Goldstein and Shelly, using similar tests, found similar selective deficiencies in ability for abstract reasoning, with relatively normal functioning in other regards (15).

Jones and Parsons, comparing hospitalized alcoholics with brain-damaged and healthy controls, also found that alcoholics manifested a deficit on the Halstead Category Test similar to that of the brain-damaged subjects. The performance deficit of the alcoholics was related positively to number of years of drinking, independent of age (16).

The alcoholics in the three studies all had IQs comparable to that of the controls. In two of the studies (14, 15) there also appeared to be impaired memory for spatial relations and impaired auditory discrimination. Language abilities remained intact.

In most studies reviewed here, alcoholics were drawn chiefly from lower middle and lower socioeconomic classes; it was often unclear whether the control groups were of comparable background.. Recognizing this, Smith *et al.* (17) studied a group of alcoholics of middle and upper socioeconomic background. The men had higher than average IQs, above average educational background, and held responsible jobs. Nevertheless, more than half showed "serious impairment" on the Category Test of the Halstead Battery. The authors interpreted this to indicate that intelligent patients with a good job history might still have trouble learning a new line of work because of loss of "capacity to deal with new problems and situations."

Unlike the results of two studies discussed below where the Trail Making Test had been administered, the men in the Smith *et al.* study did not differ from nonalcoholics in their ability to perform on this test. The Smith study had a control group but it was not clear where the controls had been obtained, since it was noted that testing was carried out at different times, at different facilities, and by different research personnel.

Trail Making Test

Fitzhugh *et al.* (14) and Goldstein and Shelly (15) combined this test with the Halstead Battery, reporting that alcoholics did less well at problem solving and had reduced psychomotor speed compared to controls. As noted by Kleinknecht and Goldstein (10), the Trail Making Test has features similar to the Digit Symbol subtest of the Wechsler Bellevue, a subtest where alcoholics frequently show impairment. As noted by Jonsson *et al.*, however, the Digit Symbol subtest is believed by many psychologists to be highly susceptible to anxiety and other disruptive affects, which may have influenced the test findings (18).

Wisconsin Card Sorting Test

Courville reported that the neuropathology of chronic alcoholism was primarily in the dorsolateral aspects of the frontal lobes with atrophy as its main characteristic (18). Milner, studying patients with dorsolateral lesions of the frontal cortex, found the Wisconsin Card Sorting Test was a sensitive instrument in registering defects in abstracting ability observed in such patients (19). Extrapolating from these observations, (*i.e.*, hypothesizing that damage to the frontal lobes of alcoholics may be responsible for their relatively poor abstracting ability), two investigations of alcoholics have been conducted using the Wisconsin Card Sorting Test. Introduced by Grant and Berg (20) in 1948, the Wisconsin Card Sorting Test was performed as follows:

> The materials consisted of a pack of four stimulus cards and 64 response cards which were devised so that each card contained from one to four identical figures of a single color. Four kinds of figures were used: stars, crosses, triangles, and circles. Four different colors were used: red, yellow, green, and blue. A single card might have four red stars, or two

> green circles, or any of the 64 possible combinations of colors, numbers, and forms. Each card could then be sorted or categorized according to the color, the number, or the form of the figure. The four stimulus cards were: first, one red triangle; second, two green stars; third, three yellow crosses; and fourth, four blue circles.
>
> The four stimulus cards were placed before the S from left to right in the order named. The S was given the pack of response cards and was instructed in the following manner: "I want you to put these cards into four groups, underneath the ones lying on the table. I will tell you whether you are "right" or "wrong."
>
> The initial 'correct' sorting category was arbitrarily determined in advance to be color. As the S sorted the response cards he was informed whether he was 'right' or 'wrong.' As soon as the S made a certain number of consecutive correct responses (reinforcing or confirming trials), the E shifted the problem with no explanation to S and began to call the number classification 'right' and all others, including color, 'wrong.' In this way, the 'correct' classification or category was later shifted from number to form, then back to number, then to color, and finally to form. The S's only cue to the shifts was in the E's 'rights' or 'wrongs.' If the S used the whole pack of cards before the six successive sorting categories were completed, the cards were reassembled and handed back to him. The cards were always presented in a standardized order so that no like form, color, or number followed each other. The experiment was considered completed after the S had finished the six categories or used more than 64 cards in a single category.

Tarter and Parsons (21) administered the Wisconsin Card Sorting Test to alcoholics and compared the results with those obtained from hospital controls and students. The alcoholics made significantly more errors. However, these differences could not be attributed to perseveration, the authors felt, but rather appeared to reflect a deficit in "sustaining a pattern of search and persistence in problem solution" on the part of the alcoholics. Duration of drinking history was related to impairment of task persistence. The authors felt that subcortical organic involvement rather than a frontal lesion, was more consistent with the difficulty in "conceptual shifting" tasks.

In a subsequent study, Tarter (22) administered the Wisconsin Card Sorting Test to alcoholics and reported that those subjects with a history of alcoholism greater than 10 years were impaired at set persistence, set shifting and error utilization when contrasted with normal controls. Alcoholics who had a history of less than 10 years of alcoholism were deficient only in set persistence. Neither group was impaired in its ability to identify simple concepts or in learning-to-learn capacity. Tarter concluded that the behavioural deficits were consistent with a frontal-limbic focus of pathology in chronic alcoholism.

Raven's Progressive Matrices

This test has been administered to alcoholics in two studies, with conflicting results. The Matrices test is a visual-spatial, non-verbal intelligence test reported to be highly correlated with the Wechsler Adult Intelligence Test. Bauer and Johnson, comparing 34 alcoholics with a matched control group of patients with "emotional disturbances," found the alcoholics did as well on the Matrices test as did the controls and somewhat better on the Wechsler Memory Scale (23). Jones, on the other hand, found that alcoholics did as well as non-alcoholic controls on a verbal intelligence test but significantly less well than the controls on the Matrices test (24). Long-term alcoholics did worse on the Matrices test than did alcoholics with a shorter history of drinking. Among the controls and short-term alcoholics, performances on the verbal and non-verbal tests were significantly correlated but were not correlated in the case of longer term alcoholics, suggesting to the author that "differential hemisphere sensitivity" to the effects of chronic alcoholism led to a "dissociation" in factors related to intellectual functioning.

Shipley-Hartford Test

Two studies (16, 24) failed to find differences in Shipley-Hartford performance between alcoholics and nonalcoholics. In another study (25), jailed alcoholics were impaired on "abstract reasoning" on the Shipley-Hartford test but had an above average vocabulary, resulting in an IQ within the average range.

Bender Gestalt Test

This well-known measure of "organicity" has been applied to two groups of alcoholics, with disparate results. Kaldegg (7) reported that 11 of 18 alcoholics did poorly on the test, although he attributed this to "neurotic" rather than organic factors. To assess the role of peripheral neuropathy in the Bender Gestalt, Hirschenfang, Silber and Benton (26) compared the drawings of alcoholics with neuropathy to drawings by subjects suffering from neuropathy of a nonalcoholic origin. There was no difference between the two groups.

METHODOLOGICAL CONSIDERATIONS

Two conclusions can tentatively be drawn from a summary of the above studies. 1. Alcoholics have normal IQs. 2. They have specific deficits in "abstracting ability," as measured by the Halstead Category Test, and in "conceptual shifting" as measured by the Wisconsin Card Sorting Test.

The latter deficits, however, apparently do not interfere with overall adaptation, at least in well-educated, intelligent individuals (17). Moreover, the data rarely bear on a vital question: are the deficits reversible?

The literature on alcoholism and organicity, in fact, is replete with instances of *reversible* cognitive impairment. To cite a few examples:

1. White (27) administered an object sorting test to a group of 50 Alcoholics Anonymous members and found that those sober from one to three months made significantly fewer "abstract-volitional shifts" than those with three years of sobriety.

2. In a study by Jonsson *et al* (28) in which a large number of intellectual function tests were administered to alcoholics, it was found that performances were worse in the group that was examined at the beginning of the term in hospital than in the group examined at the end. In only two tests, Wechsler's Digit Symbol and Grassi's Block Substitution Test, was there no evidence of restitution by the end of hospitalization. Jonsson *et al.* concluded that "the general trend suggests a partially reversible impairment of intellectual ability immediately after a period of intensive abuse of alcohol."

3. Plumeau *et al.* (6) compared alcoholics in remission (at least two years abstinent) with unremitted alcoholics and found the latter group had poorer test results than controls and the remitted cases. Both alcoholic groups were "identical as regard to the duration and intensity of alcoholism." An analysis of WAIS subscales revealed no differences between the remitted alcoholics and normal controls.

4. Smith and Layden (29) showed improvement in perceptual motor function after prolonged abstinence from alcohol, comparing alcoholics during and after hospital treatment.

5. Bennett (30), in a study of 227 alcoholics, found abnormal electroencephalograms in 139. After several months of abstinence, many of the records returned to normal.

6. Goldstein (31) showed that gait instability in alcoholics was reversible and that practice potentiates the degree of improvement.

7. Smith *et al.* (25) administered tests to alcoholics soon after admission and again after two weeks. Significant improvement was found on the second testing with regard to Shipley-Hartford measures of vocabulary and abstract reasoning, the Embedded Figures Test and the Hidden Figures Test.

8. Weingartner *et al.* (32) and Allen *et al.* (33) demonstrated a post-binge syndrome which included a learning deficit attributable to an impairment in holding information in memory or storage. This Korsakoff-like deficit disappeared after three weeks of abstinence in the hospital.

9. Witkin *et al.* (34) reported that alcoholics were more "field dependent" than nonalcoholics, but Goldstein and Chotlos (35) reported they became more "field independent" after a period of abstinence.

10. In a study recently conducted in our department (36), it was found that 8 of 16 newly admitted alcoholics manifested "organicity" on a test developed by Canter (37-39) based on a modification of the Bender Gestalt Test. The test involves redrawing the Bender designs on paper that has a light background of wavy lines. In patients with brain damage this background apparently "interferes" with the ability to reproduce the Bender design and the test has been called the Bender Interference Procedure (BIP). Although the test has been well validated as a measure of chronic brain damage (40), it was found the "brain damaged" alcoholics improved significantly in their performance on the test after one month in the hospital. (A longer follow-up is planned to determine whether the impairment is completely reversible over a period of several months or longer.)

The above examples illustrate the importance of separating acute from chronic effects of alcohol, and the difficulties in doing this by studying recently hospitalized patients. The evidence is strong that at least some of the deficits from abuse of alcohol are indeed reversible, and it is possible that even the consistently shown deficits in "abstracting ability" and "conceptual shifts" may be reversible over time.

Alcoholism is undoubtedly associated with permanent brain pathology, but in the most studied example of this, *i.e.*, Korsakoff's syndrome, the etiology has been definitely shown to be nutritional, based on a specific thiamine deficiency (41). The cerebellar degenerative lesions associated with alcoholism are less well demonstrated to be nutritional in origin, but many authorities believe this is probably the case. Peripheral neuropathy associated with alcoholism, again, is almost certainly due to vitamin deficiency and is almost always reversible, if treated early (41).

Post-mortem findings of cortical atrophy in alcoholics will be discussed elsewhere, as well as the pneumoencephalographic and electroencephalographic evidence of brain damage. Even if the association of atrophy and alcoholism is confirmed beyond a doubt (which, in the author's opinion, has not been done), it still could not be definitely concluded that alcohol *per se* was the offending agent.

Complicating the interpretation of all of the medical and neurological illnesses associated with alcoholism is the fact that alcoholics are usually malnourished, are almost universally heavy smokers, are frequently subject to head trauma, and differ from other groups in their habits and life style. Furthermore, alcoholics rarely drink pure ethyl alcohol but usually alcoholic *beverages* rich in congeners, including the "higher" alcohols known to be particularly toxic.

In vitro studies, with the exception of those by Tewari and Noble (42), have been inconclusive with respect to the neurotoxicity of ethanol itself.

Other methodological difficulties in separating acute from chronic effects of alcohol have been reviewed by Kleinknecht and Goldstein (10), and include the following:

1. Commonly, in studies of intellectual functioning during the immediate post-admission period, patients receive a variety of psychotropic medications, and this may contribute to impaired test performance.

2. Many studies lack an appropriate control group with matching by age, race, education, and other demographic variables. Test results in most instruments are influenced by age, and having even a few older alcoholics in the experimental group may skew the results.

3. Motivation is an important variable in performing most tests. Recently hospitalized alcoholics, often heavily medicated and despondent about their situation, might conceivably be less motivated to cooperate in testing than individuals hospitalized for other reasons, or than healthy controls.

Also, it may be important whether the subjects are volunteers or nonvolunteers. Cox and Sipprelle (43) found that volunteer-nonvolunteer status was an important variable in determining the results of a heart-rate conditioning experiment. If a conditioning experiment can be thus influenced, the importance of motivation in taking a battery of psychological tests is obvious.

Another difficulty in evaluating chronic effects of alcohol on intellectual functioning pertains to distinguishing cause from consequence. Kaij (44), for example, administered a series of cognitive tests to twin pairs where one of the twins was alcoholic. He found that "deterioration" was more correlated with zygosity than with extent of drinking; *i.e.*, a "deteriorated" heavy drinking monozygotic twin was more likely to have a light drinking partner showing signs of deterioration than was true of dizygotic twins where one partner was deteriorated. He interpreted this as indicating that so-called "alcoholic deterioration" occurred more or less independently of alcohol consumption and may be a genetically determined contributor to the illness rather than a consequence.

The difficulty of alcoholics in "adapting" after they have stopped drinking is often attributed to permanent effects on brain function from years of heavy drinking (14, 18). Longitudinal studies are needed to show whether adaptive difficulties precede as well as follow the drinking history. The psychological tests which are apparently most sensitive to organicity in alcoholics, namely, the Halstead Category Test and the Wisconsin Card Sorting Test, have not been administered to alcoholics before they become alcoholic. Since the children of alcoholics are at particularly high risk for developing alcoholism themselves, a worthwhile study would be to administer these tests to the offspring of alcoholics to determine whether they perform more poorly than a matched control group. Perhaps poor "conceptual shifting" is a cause rather than a result of heavy drinking.

A number of investigators, ignoring the difficulty in distinguishing acute and subacute effects from chronic effects of alcohol, have suggested that one effect of alcoholism is premature senescence. Intellectual functioning tends to decline with increasing age and several studies have suggested that younger alcoholics resemble aging nonalcoholics in their test performances (9, 14, 16). These theories to some extent reflect the influence of Courville (18) who stated categorically that alcohol "hastened and accentuated the aging process to the end that the body and brain of the habituated individual become prematurely old."

Evidence that this "aging" may be reversible is generally overlooked. Smith *et al.* (25) reported that alcoholics had an electroencephalographic sleep pattern resembling that of older persons where delta sleep is relatively absent – evidence, they believed, of "diffuse cortical damage." A recent study, however, of alcoholics dry for a year or longer showed a relatively normal sleep pattern for the subjects' age (45).

In summary, alcoholism unquestionably is associated with brain damage, Korsakoff's syndrome being the classic example. Its association with permanently impaired intellectual functioning is more equivocal, principally because of the paucity of studies of alcoholics who have stopped drinking for long periods of time and the likely confusion of acute with chronic effects. Moreover, to the extent it exists, the association is with *alcoholism* rather than with alcohol.

Alcoholism is a clinical syndrome characterized not only by excessive consumption of alcohol but also by malnutrition, a high instance of head trauma, heavy smoking, liver disease, other medical complications, and usually a highly irregular life style. Some indirect evidence (42, 46) does suggest that alcohol may have a permanent effect on brain function, but this evidence is more anatomical and biochemical than based on clinical observation or psychological tests.

Indeed, it is impressive how *well* alcoholics perform on psychological tests, given all of the potentially harmful influences noted above. Even after many years of very heavy drinking, alcoholics show little objective evidence of brain damage, *provided* a sufficiently long period has passed between the last drink and time of testing. It is generally believed that residual effects from heavy drinking (especially insomnia) may persist for at least several months, and, before an alcoholic is said to have permanent brain damage, at least a period of that interval should have passed before observations are made (47). Even then, it may be incorrect to say his impairment came "from" drinking since the drinking is often accompanied by so many other pathologic influences.

DRUG STUDIES

Compared to the alcoholism literature, there have been relatively few studies regarding possible chronic effects of what today are referred to as "psychotropic" drugs. Precisely the same problems apply to these studies as were described above under methodological issues: the problem of reversibility, cause-and-effect, test design, etc. In addition, drug studies are complicated by a factor presumably less important in alcohol studies: drug users commonly use a variety of drugs and it is often difficult if not impossible to parcel out the effects of individual drugs.

Nevertheless, several investigators have attempted to determine whether two drugs, LSD and marihuana, if used frequently, have adverse permanent effects on intellectual functioning.

Several animal studies suggest that LSD may produce pathological changes in the brain. Denber *et al.* (48) reported that single doses of 25 mg/kg of body weight injected into the rat were associated with loss of nuclear chromatin in neurones. The effect was not observed with 1 mg/kg. Sharpe *et al.* (49) reported that squirrel monkeys given 10 mcg/kg of LSD for five days sustained a disruption of size discrimination if the task was difficult but not if the task was easy. The effect persisted for months after the last injection. Adey (50) reported that LSD produced post-injection alteration of hippocampal electrographic patterns for days to weeks in monkeys.

In 1968 Kiely (51) described a "slippage" in "logical thought processes" and other defects in cognitive function in five teenagers who had been on more than 50 LSD trips. The defects were subtle and poorly defined.

In the first well-controlled study of possible chronic effects from LSD, Cohen and Edwards (52) compared 30 young men and women who had used LSD 50 or more times with 30 control subjects matched for sex, age, educational and socioeconomic background, where the controls had no experience with LSD. Tests administered included the Halstead Battery, the Trail Making A Test, and the Raven's Progressive Matrices.

The LSD users differed from controls in that they did significantly worse on the Raven's Spatial-Orientation Test and on the Trail Making Test. Ranked with regard to the number of times they had used LSD, the more frequent users had significantly lower IQs, although, as the authors pointed out, it was possible that less intelligent persons tended to use LSD more often. Frequency of use was also positively correlated with poor performance on the Trails test but not with performance on the Raven's test.

The spatially oriented task involves following a visually presented map. The Trail Making task involves successive searchings through space for a destination. Both, as the authors point out, involve learning as well as neurological intactness. Conceivably, frequent experience with a spatially disorienting drug such as LSD could result in partial loss of a previously learned technique, which might explain why none of the other tests showed impairment.

Data were also collected on drugs other than LSD used by the subjects. None was correlated with any test result. The authors tentatively concluded that while there was no evidence of a generalized psychoneurological dysfunction attributable to taking LSD at least 50 times, there was evidence of impairment of visual spatial orientation, and the inverse relationship between general intelligence and number of LSD exposures warranted further study.

Blacker *et al.* (53) administered a series of cognitive tasks to 21 chronic LSD users. Interpretation of the results was complicated by great variability among members of the group, some of whom performed as well as normal subjects. The authors concluded that heavy LSD usage was compatible with normal performance but that "a number of our LSD users were slow."

The LSD users, as a group, did differ from a control group on a visual evoked response measure and this, plus abnormal EEG findings, suggested "minimal brain damage." The authors stressed, however, that the evidence for this was "scattered and inconclusive, particularly in the absence of consistent abnormal psychological test findings."

McGlothlin *et al.* (54) compared 16 regular LSD users with 16 non-LSD controls. The test battery included the two tests which differentiated the LSD group in the Cohen and Edwards (52) study, namely, the Trail Making A Test and the Spatial Orientation Test. The former measures the speed with which the subject can scan a series of randomly scattered circles numbered 1 to 25, and correct them in sequence. The second requires the subject to walk out a visually presented map which he holds in a constant fashion with respect to himself. This task is similar to following a street map without orienting the map to match the geographic coordinates.

In addition the subjects were given the Porteus Maze and several other tasks, including the Witkins Embedded Figures Test and tests from the Halstead Battery.

Only one measure, the Halstead Category Test, yielded significant differences between the two groups. The mean number of errors made by the LSD group was larger beyond the .01 level of confidence. The LSD group also obtained a somewhat lower score on the abstract portion of the Shipley-Hartford, which is similar to the Category Test. Neither of the tests which differentiated the LSD and comparison groups in the Cohen and Edwards study – Trail Making A and Spatial Orientation – showed significant differences in the McGlothlin study. Both, however, did show poorer scores for the LSD group, and the difference for Trail Making A approached significance.

The LSD and control groups had similar IQs and there was no evidence of generalized organicity in the LSD group. Even on the Category Test, on which the LSD group showed the poorest performance, the mean number of errors was considerably short of the mean score norms obtained by persons with proven brain damage (55). However, the authors concluded there was at least some evidence of organicity. The relatively poor performance on the Category Test coupled with high scores on verbal measures was consistent with the "well established" observation that abstract abilities are more impaired by CNS damage than are verbal abilities, and the Category Test was described as the "most sensitive subtest in the Halstead Battery for detecting organicity."

Acord and Barker (56) studied 30 subjects from the inpatient and outpatient services and staff of a large military hospital. Half of them, on at least one occasion, had ingested an hallucinogenic drug (LSD, STP, DMT, mescaline, or psilocybin). The controls denied using hallucinogenic drugs, although most had used marihuana. All were administered three tests previously found to be "sensitive to cerebral damage." These were taken from the Indiana Neuropsychological Battery and included the Tactal Performance Test, localization; the Trail Making Test part B; and the Category Test from the Halstead Battery.

Subjects who had used hallucinogenic drugs performed significantly less well than did controls on the Trail Making Test and the Category Test. Using Halstead's and Reitan's cut-off scores, all of the drug subjects scored in the brain-damaged range on at least one of the three tests, whereas only seven of the controls did so. The authors concluded there was evidence of impairment of "highest level abstraction ability" associated with drug use.

In summary, four studies have indicated selective intellectual functioning deficits in chronic users of LSD, although all of the investigators caution against premature interpretation of actual brain damage. Similar caution has been urged with regard to two studies in which drug users appear to differ from normal controls in electroencephalographic readings (57) and pneumoencephalography (58). Both studies concluded there was a significant dilation of the third ventricle when drug users were compared with normal controls. Both studies involved polydrug users and neither had a formal control group.

Although marihuana has been used much more extensively than LSD and other hallucinogenic drugs, even less is known about possible chronic effects on intellectual functioning. Grant *et al.* (59) recently compared 29 medical students who had smoked marihuana more than 50 times with 29 non-users. The subjects were administered the Halstead Category Test, the Tactal Performance Test, Reitan's Trail Making Test, Raven's Progressive Matrices, and the Goal Directed Serial Alternation Test. No difference was found between the smokers and nonsmokers on seven of the eight measures. The smokers did perform less well on three subtests of the Tactal Performance Test, but the authors felt this probably had no significance. Their results agreed with those of Mendelson and Meyer (60) who employed similar tests with 10 casual and 10 heavy users.

Entin and Goldzung (61) used paired associate learning lists to test memory and acquisition of new information in students, half of whom had smoked marihuana daily for at least six months, with a matched control group of nonsmokers. Neither group smoked marihuana on the day of the experiment. Despite being unintoxicated, the marihuana users had significantly more difficulty both with respect to memory and acquiring new learning. A mathematical task later was administered and there was no significant difference between smokers and nonsmokers.

The authors concluded the difference between the verbal and numerical task results may have been attributable to the shorter memory interval involved in the numerical task. They also studied the effect of other drugs, "test anxiety," and academic ability as possible confounding variables in the differences in verbal learning between smokers and nonsmokers, and concluded that none of these influenced the results.

Because the user and nonuser groups were comparable in academic achievement, the authors concluded the memory impairment had little deleterious effect on the smokers' overall intellectual functioning. Also, since the test occurred shortly after a long period of a daily smoking, even minimal "hangover" effects may have impaired performance in the smoker group.

One difficulty in evaluating chronic effects from marihuana among American users is that the drug has been used for a relatively short period in this country and often has been of low potency. Studies of foreign populations of chronic cannabis users are now under way in an effort to provide more information about chronic effects without having to wait many years before our own chronic users become appropriate subjects for study.

One study is being conducted in Greece where chronic hashish users have been subjected to intensive medical, neurological and psychiatric study. The average years of use in the group was 27. So far, there has been no evidence of significant neurological signs or symptoms in the group and none has had an organic brain syndrome. EEG records have generally been normal.

Another study is being conducted in Jamaica, matching nonuser controls with chronic cannabis users. Each group consists of 30 individuals. Ninety percent of the users were daily smokers. Again, intensive medical, neurological, psychological, and psychiatric investigations have shown little evidence of differences between the two groups.

In making available these preliminary findings, the National Institute of Mental Health emphasized their preliminary nature and the importance of waiting for a complete analysis of the results (62).

At any rate, at this time there exists no well-controlled investigation linking chronic marihuana use to permanent effects on intellectual functioning; and, as is the case of all drugs reviewed in this paper (including alcohol), in no instance have acute effects been sufficiently delineated from chronic effects to permit definite conclusions about the latter.

ACKNOWLEDGEMENTS

This work was supported, in part, by U.S.P.H.S. Grant MH09247 and a Research Scientist Development Award MH47325 from the National Institute of Mental Health (Dr. Goodwin).

REFERENCES

1. Wechsler D: The Measurement and Appraisal of Adult Intelligence. Fourth edition. Baltimore, Williams & Wilkins, 1958
2. Robins L, Davis D, Goodwin D: Unpublished data.
3. Halpern F: Studies of compulsive drinkers; psychological test results. Quart J Stud Alc 6: 468-479, 1946
4. Murphy MM: Social class differences in intellectual characteristics of alcoholics. Quart J Stud Alc 14: 192-196, 1953
5. Peters GA Jr: Emotional and intellectual concomitants of advanced chronic alcoholism. J Cons Psychol 20: 390, 1956
6. Plumeau F, Machover S, Puzzo F: Wechsler-Bellevue performances of remitted and unremitted alcoholics, and their normal controls. J Cons Psychol 24: 240-242, 1960

7. Kaldegg A: Psychological observation in a group of alcoholic patients; with analysis of Rorschach, Wechsler-Bellevue and Bender Gestalt test results. Quart J Stud Alc 17: 608-628, 1956
8. Teicher MI, Singer EA: A report on the use of the W-B scales in an overseas general hospital. Amer J Psychiat 103: 91-93, 1946
9. Fitzhugh KB, Fitzhugh LC, Reitan RM: Wechsler-Bellevue comparisons in groups of "chronic" and "current" lateralized and diffuse brain lesions. J Cons Psychol 26: 306-310, 1962
10. Kleinknecht RA, Goldstein SG: Neuropsychological deficits associated with alcoholism. Quart J Stud Alc 33: 999-1019, 1972
11. Klebanoff SG, Singer JL, Wilensky H: Psychological consequences of brain lesions and ablations. Psychol Bull 51: 1-41, 1954
12. Morrow RS, Mark JC: Correlation of intelligence and neurological findings on 22 patients autopsied for brain damage. Am J Psychol 9: 435, 1954
13. Wittenborn JR: An evaluation of the Wechsler-Bellevue subtest scores as an aid in psychiatric diagnosis. J Cons Psychol 13: 433-439, 1949
14. Fitzhugh LC, Fitzhugh KB, Reitan RM: Adaptive abilities and intellectual functioning of hospitalized alcoholics; further considerations. Quart J Stud Alc 26: 402-411, 1965
15. Goldstein G, Shelly CH: Field dependence and cognitive, perceptual and motor skills in alcoholics. Quart J Stud Alc 32: 29-40, 1971
16. Jones B, Parsons OA: Impaired abstracting ability in chronic alcoholics. Arch Gen Psychiat 24: 71-75, 1971
17. Smith JW, Burt DW, Chapman RF: Intelligence and brain damage in alcoholics. Quart J Stud Alc 34: 414-422, 1973
18. Courville CB: Effects of Alcohol on the nervous System of Man. Los Angeles, San Lucas, 1955
19. Milner B: Effects of different brain lesions on card sorting. Arch Neurol 9: 90-100, 1963
20. Grant DA, Berg EA: A behavioral analysis of degree of reinforcement and ease of shifting to new responses in a weigl-type card sorting problem. J Exp Psychol 38: 404-411, 1948
21. Tarter R, Parsons O: Conceptual shifting in chronic alcoholics. J Abnorm Psychol 77: 71-75, 1971
22. Tarter RE: An analysis of cognitive deficits in chronic alcoholics. J Nerv Ment Dis 157: 138-147, 1973
23. Bauer RW, Johnson DE: The question of deterioration in alcoholism. J Cons Psychol 21: 296, 1957
24. Jones BM: Verbal and spatial intelligence in short and long term alcoholics. J Nerv Ment Dis 153: 292-297, 1971
25. Smith JW, Johnson LC, Burdick JA: Sleep, psychological and clinical changes during alcohol withdrawal in NAD-treated alcoholics. Quart J Stud Alc 32: 982-994, 1971
26. Hirschenfang S, Silber M, Benton JG: Comparison of Bender Gestalt reproductions by patients with peripheral neuropathy. Percept Motor Skills 24: 1317-1318, 1967
27. White WF: Personality and cognitive learning among alcoholics with different intervals of sobriety. Psychol Rep 16: 1125-1140, 1965
28. Jonsson CO, Cronholm B, Izikowitz S: Intellectual changes in alcoholics. Quart J Stud Alc 23: 221-242, 1962
29. Smith JW, Layden TA: Changes in psychological performance and blood chemistry in alcoholics during and after hospital treatment. Quart J Stud Alc 33: 379-394, 1972
30. Bennett AE: Diagnosis of intermediate stage of alcoholic brain disease. J Amer Med Assoc 172: 1143-1146, 1960
31. Goldstein G. Chotlos JW, McCarthy RJ, et al: Recovery from gait instability in alcoholics. Quart J Stud Alc 29: 38-43, 1968
32. Weingartner H, Faillace LA, Markley HG: Verbal information retention in alcoholics. Quart J Stud Alc 32: 293-303, 1971
33. Allen RP, Faillace LA, Reynolds DM: Recovery of memory functioning in alcoholics following prolonged alcohol intoxication. J Nerv Ment Dis 153: 417-423, 1971
34. Witkin HA, Karp SA, Goodenough DR: Dependence in alcoholics. Quart J Stud Alc 20: 493-504, 1959

35. Goldstein G. Chotlos JW: Stability of field dependence in chronic alcoholic patients. J Abnorm Psychol 71: 420, 1966
36. Hill SY, Goodwin DW: Unpublished data
37. Canter A: A background interference procedure for graphomotor tests in the study of deficit. Percept Motor Skills 16: 914, 1963
38. Canter A: A background interference procedure to increase sensitivity of the Bender-Gestalt test to organic brain damage. J Consult Psychol 30: 91-97, 1966
39. Canter A: The BIP-Bender Test for the detection of organic brain disorder: Modified scoring method and replication. J Consult Clin Psychol 32: 522-526, 1968
40. Yulis S: Performance of normal and organic brain damaged subjects on the Canter Background Interference Procedure Test as a function of drive. J Consult Clin Psychol 34: 184-188, 1970
41. Victor M, Adams RD, Collins GH: The Wernicke-Korsakoff Syndrome. Philadelphia, F. A. Davis Company, 1971
42. Tewari S, Noble EP: Ethanol and brain protein synthesis. Brain Research 26: 469-474, 1971
43. Cox DE, Sipprelle CN: Coercion in participation as a research subject. Amer Psychologist 26: 726-728, 1971
44. Kaij L: Alcoholism in Twins. Stockholm, Almqvist and Wiksell, 1960.
45. Adamson J, Burdick JA: Sleep of dry alcoholics. Arch Gen Psychiat 28: 146-149, 1973
46. Moskow HA, Pennington RC, Knisely MH: Alcohol, sludge, and hypoxic areas of nervous system, liver and heart. Microvasc Res 1: 174-185, 1968
47. Johnson L, Slye E, Dement W: EEG and autonomic activity during and after prolonged sleep deprivation. Psychosom Med, 1965
48. Denber HCB, Charipper HA, Roizen L: Cytological effects of lysergic acid diethylamide in rat brain and liver. Fed Proc 23: 147, 1964
49. Sharpe LG, Otis LS, Schusterman RJ: Disruption of size discrimination in squirrel monkeys (Saimiri Saureus) by LSD-25. Psychon Sci 7, 3: 103-104, 1967
50. Adey WR et al: Prolonged effects of LSD on EEG records during discriminative performance in cat: Evaluation by computer analysis. Electroenceph Clin Neurophysiol 18: 25-35, 1965
51. Kiely WF: Paper presented at the 49th annual meeting of the Americal College of Physicians, Boston, Mass April 1-5, 1968
52. Cohen S, Edwards AE: LSD and organic brain impairment. Read before the Section on Nervous and Mental Diseases, American Medical Association, San Francisco, California, June 18, 1968
53. Blacker KH, Jones RT, Stone GC et al: Chronic users of LSD: The "acidheads." Amer J Psychiat 125: 97-107, 1968
54. McGlothlin WH, Arnold DO, Freedman DX: Organicity measures following repeated LSD ingestion. Arch Gen Psychiat 21: 704-709, 1969
55. Halstead WC: Brain and Intelligence. Chicago, Univ. Chicago Press, 1947
56. Acord LD, Barker DD: Hallucinogenic drugs and cerebral deficit. J Nerv Ment Dis 156: 281-283, 1973
57. Von Zerssen D, Fliege K, Wolf M: Cerebral atrophy in drug addicts. Lancet 2: 313, 1970
58. Campbell AMG, Evans M, Thomson JLG et al: Cerebral atrophy in young cannabis smokers. Lancet 2: 341-351, 1968
59. Grant I, Rochford J, Fleming T et al: A neuropsychological assessment of the effects of moderate marihuana use. J Nerv Ment Dis 156: 278-280, 1973
60. Mendelson JH, Meyer RE: Behavioral and biological concomitants of chronic marihuana smoking by heavy and casual users. In Technical Papers of the First Report of the National Commission on Marihuana and Drug Abuse, pp. 68-246. U.S. Government Printing Office, Washington, D.C., 1972
61. Entin EE, Goldzung PJ: Residual effects of marihuana usage on learning and memory. Psychol Rec 23: 169-178, 1973
62. Marihuana and Health. Second Annual Report to Congress from The Secretary of Health, Education, and Welfare, 1972

Long-Term Behavioural Consequences of Exposure to Drugs and Pollutants

Bernard Weiss

The issues with which this paper deals currently pervade the disciplines of toxicology and environmental health. The most troublesome problems they face revolve about the consequences of long-term exposure to chemicals at levels low enough not to produce clear poisoning. That is, they center on the question of subclinical damage.

Behavioural toxicology assumes a special role in these problems. In the first place, many substances act primarily on the central nervous system, exerting directly mediated effects. Heavy metals and organic solvents are examples of substances that fall into this category. In the second place, an even more numerous collection of chemicals can produce vague, nonspecific complaints early in intoxication, before the overt signs appear. Such complaints possess a large psychological component.

Behavioural assessments are particularly useful in ambiguous situations because behaviour is a reflection of total organism functioning. They can help to determine when compensatory mechanisms are no longer able to counteract some toxic effect whose progress has obliterated the excess functional capacity of a particular system.

When we discuss the long term consequences of chemicals that serve no useful therapeutic purpose we seek to define exposure levels that minimize risks to the exposed population. Our estimates of dose are deliberately conservative. When we deal with chemicals employed as therapeutic agents, we tend to accept a much higher incidence of toxic reactions and greater risks to health.

Whatever we choose to accept is governed then, by balancing risks against benefits. I want to address the evaluation of hazards over the long term, with special reference to what might be called *temporal drift* in their constellation.

THERAPEUTIC AGENTS

We all know that drugs are not free of actions apart from the therapeutic aim for which they are chosen. When such actions become apparent early in the course of therapy, countervailing measures can be taken, including the cessation of therapy. When such countermeasures are not taken, or when a long latency supervenes, they present a special danger, because, by that time, a relatively large population may have been exposed (for example, the case of stilbesterol and vaginal cancer). A cogent example from psychopharmacology is the class of agents known as the major tranquilizers, especially the phenothiazines and butyrophenones.

When the phenothiazines first were introduced for the chemical treatment of behaviour disorders, significant numbers of patients were observed to develop symptoms of extrapyramidal disorders, a syndrome that clinicians termed pseudo-Parkinsonism. This phenomenon is perhaps the best known toxic action of phenothiazine therapy.

A more recently recognized concomitant of major tranquilizer therapy is the so-called tardive dyskinesia (1). After a relatively extended period of treatment, a certain proportion of patients, sometimes estimated to be the majority, display what seem to be irreversible symptoms. The most consistent are mouth and jaw movements, but other kinds of movement disorders also appear. At the same time that these drugs may be responsible for the problem, they also may be the source of therapy. At sufficiently high doses they apparently manage to suppress the dyskinesia, and patients returned to the drug after withdrawal may show diminutions in these reactions (2, 3).

Haloperidol, a butyrophenone widely used in Europe for the treatment of behaviour disorders, is one of the most potent of these agents. Earlier observations in this laboratory by Dr. Tina Levine, of squirrel monkeys (*s. sciurea*) chronically maintained on haloperidol, induced us to attempt a long term study in a cebus monkey (*c. apella*). This animal, a mature female, has now been receiving the drug orally for eight months.

The haloperidol is given orally with juice during the late morning. The monkey consumes the juice in just a few minutes. The dose is 0.5 mg/kg, which lies within but near the top of the human dose range (4).

During the early months, the typical pattern induced by the drug was sedation followed by sleep within two to four hours after drug consumption. Before it assumed a sleeping position, the monkey often displayed a variety of movements suggesting proprioceptive and visual disorientation. In the morning, it typically displayed a pattern of hyperactivity dominated by circling movements within the cage.

With continued administration, the response gradually changed in character. After about five months, instead of sedating the monkey two to four hours after ingestion, haloperidol now produced a striking picture of loss of motor control. The monkey underwent what appeared to be convulsions, flinging itself about the cage, striking the walls, assuming bizarre postures, shrieking wildly, and grasping at objects within the cage. The same pattern persists, except perhaps for a shorter latency to the violent activity and a more exaggerated response. We are planning both to instrument these kinds of reactions and to carry out a dose-response study with other cebus monkeys. Figure 1 shows some of the postures that the monkey assumes during this period. All three photographs are taken from a single period. These observations have been documented much more clearly in a motion picture film.

The change in response which we observed and that is depicted so strikingly in the film is not dissimilar to the gradual encroachment of the tardive dyskinesia syndrome. Whether the underlying CNS processes represent a process such as supersensitivity, or an alternative process, they still reflect the fact that prolonged exposure may produce qualitatively different effects than over the short term.

ENVIRONMENTAL AGENTS

Environmental contaminants offer similar problems over the long term. The problems are complicated, however, by the greater subtlety of the questions that arise. Although the therapeutic situation usually involves the simultaneous administration of many drugs, their use can be monitored and documented, more or less, and doses altered to reduce undesirable effects. It is not possible to perform the same kinds of continuous experimentation with environmental contaminants because of their often ubiquitous nature. For this reason, their effects are more likely to progress to irreversible states.

Heavy metal poisoning is an example of such a process. The intoxication often begins insidiously and tends to develop slowly. By the time clear symptoms have blossomed into visibility the damage already has been done. Manganese intoxication illustrates such a progression. Manganese poisoning is an occupational hazard for manganese miners and workers in ferro-manganese processing plants. Although the progression is not invariable, the early symptoms tend to be behavioural, at first comprising apathy and weakness, then encompassing euphoria, compulsiveness, insomnia, irritability and restlessness, a tendency to weep, and hallucinations. In the South American mining communities where manganism is well known, this syndrome is called *"locura manganica"* ("manganese madness") (5).

These early symptoms are followed by overt neurological dysfunction closely resembling Parkinsonism in its extrapyramidal character. In fact, the efficacy of L-Dopa was convincingly demonstrated here by Cotzias and his coworkers (6). With the appearance of the overt neurological signs many of the other behavioural symptoms fade. This suggests multiple system involvement or, perhaps, the destruction or inactivation within the basal ganglia of enough dopamine receptors for some other mechanism to eliminate these early behavioural symptoms and to convert them, as it were, into neurological ones.

Metallic mercury offers a very similar sequence. Again, intoxication is primarily a central nervous system phenomenon and its early manifestations are primarily psychological. In fact, these non-specific symptoms – fatigue, lassitude, irritability, a range of anxieties about the victim's functioning – are reminiscent of what psychiatrists used to call "neurasthenia". In the mercury literature, this collection of symptoms goes by the name *erethism*. Listen to this collection of complaints from a worker employed in the felt hat industry, in which inorganic mercurials were used to soften and curl the fur from which the hats were made (7):

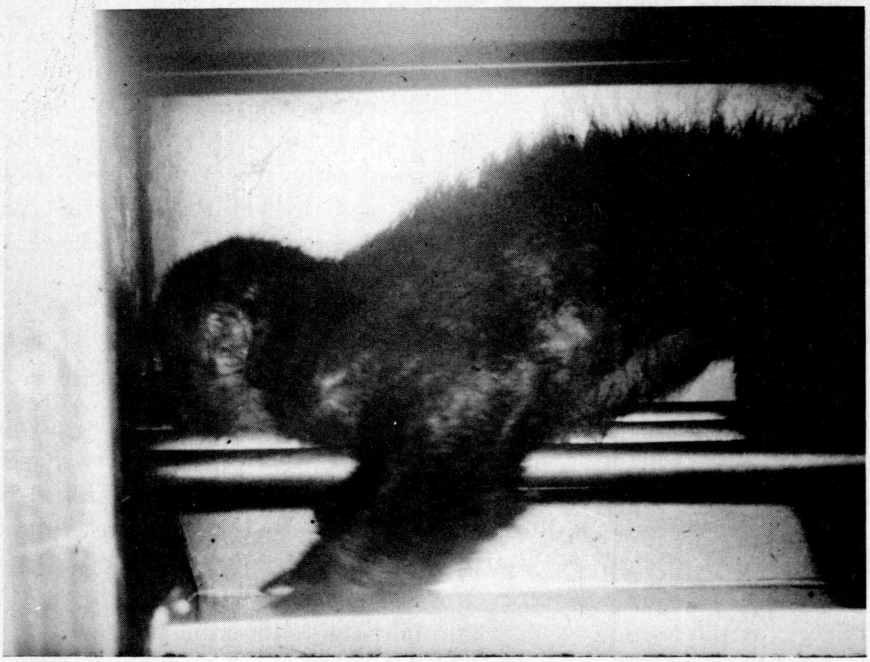

Figure 1a

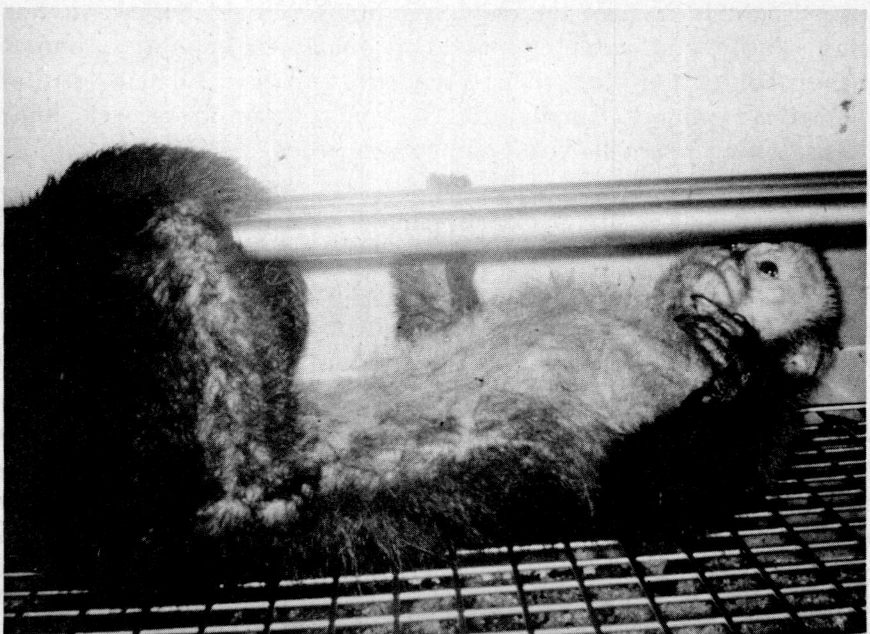

Figure 1b

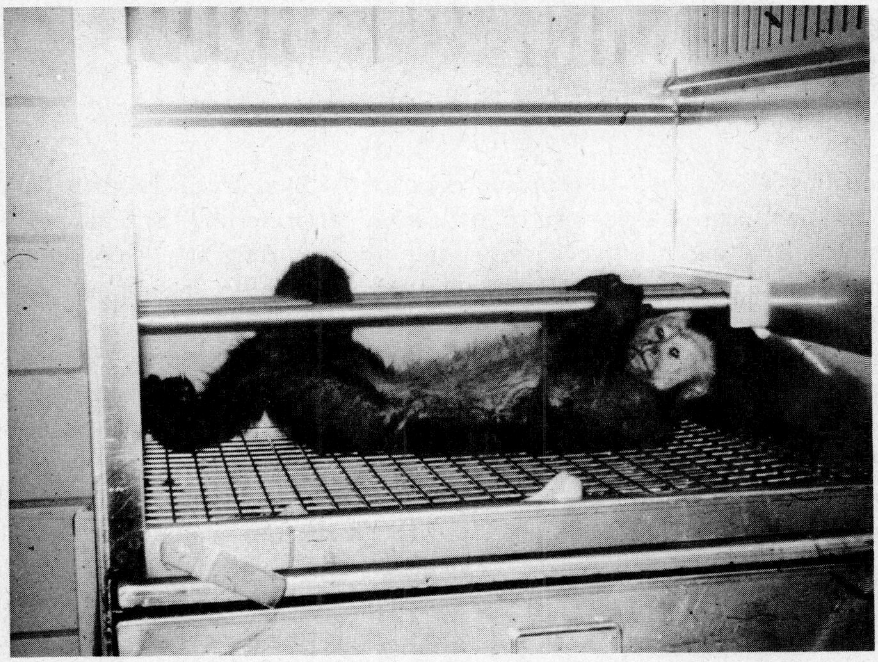

Figure 1c

Figure 1. *Three photographs taken during period of peak response to haloperidol, approximately 4 hours after oral dose of 0.5 mg/kg, 186 days after start of chronic dosing. The photographs demonstrate some of the peculiar postures assumed by the monkey during this time. Note that the monkey was not quiescent; clonic limb movements were occurring. These were interspersed with rather violent movements of the entire body.*

> . . .people get on my nerves quickly. I know that this is due to mercury poisoning and I try to control myself. . .I worry about small things, also about my work unnecessarily. . .I feel low in spirit and feel that I am not doing as well as I should.

As intoxication continues, more pronounced effects appear. The most prominent is tremor, so characteristic that it was known as "hatter's shakes." With higher exposure levels, and longer durations, the neurological impairment becomes severe, and is characterized by full-blown ataxia and other coordination deficits.

Metallic mercury is relatively benign compared to the alkyl compounds of mercury. Once exposure ends, the symptoms start to fade and the neurological impairment, at least, eventually disappears. The alkyl mercurials produce effects that seem far more permanent, much less reversible, and considerably more debilitating. This is particularly true of methylmercury, the form present in fish.

LONG-TERM CONSEQUENCES

The questions arising from the presence of methylmercury in foodstuffs, at levels too low in most parts of the world to instigate overt poisoning (8), induced us to try to consider in a quantitative fashion the possible long range consequences of exposure to such a potent central nervous system poison (9). Therapeutic agents can be viewed from a similar perspective.

Some time ago, Kety (10) tried to draw together the then available data on the relationship between age and brain function. His conclusions are shown by the heavy line in Figure 2. It depicts a decline in brain functional capacity, as measured by the indices of neuronal cell density, oxygen uptake, and blood flow, of about 20 to 25% between the ages of 25 and 75. That is, assuming that the brain functions at 100% of its capacity at age 25, there is a decline through the rest of the life span of about one-fourth. We took Kety's figures and made extrapolations on the basis of the following considerations. Suppose the individual is exposed to an environmental contaminant or a drug whose effect is to accelerate the "natural" loss in brain functional capacity. On the chart are plotted additional decrements of 0.1%, 0.5% and 1% per year. Even with an added loss of only 0.1% per year, by the time the individual is 65 years old that individual's brain is, say, 9 years older.

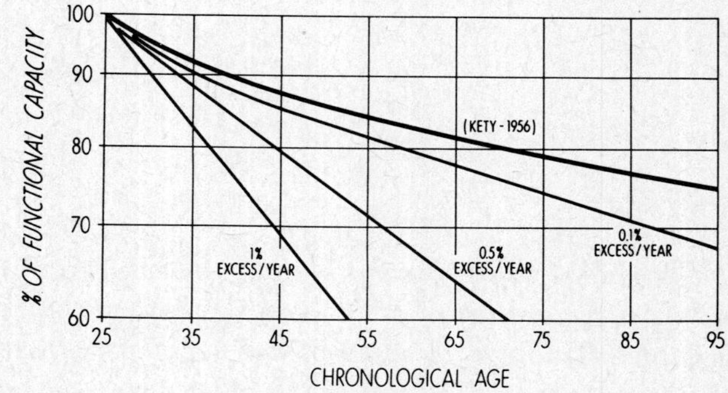

Figure 2. *Extrapolations from function proposed by Kety (10) to depict brain aging. Additional decrements of 0.1, 0.5 and 1% per year assumed. Age 25 is the baseline.*

A second view of these measures is seen in Figure 3, which depicts brain age directly as a function of chronological age, given different added accelerations in loss. Note how a loss increment of only 1% per year leads to a quite rapid ageing of the brain compared to the normal rate. We have no way to measure such a loss reliably in its early stages.

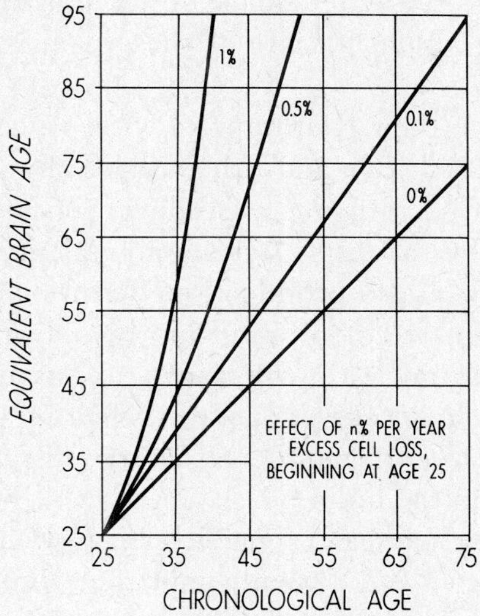

Figure 3. *Equivalent brain age given accelerations of 0.1, 0.5 and 1% per year in cell loss from age 25 to specified chronological age.*

Let me insert some warnings. I am not proposing these graphs as a model for brain ageing. Nor do I contend that methylmercury produces such an effect. Furthermore, I am not even certain that the decline as depicted by Kety and others does exist, or that it promotes any significant difference in performance. We all know of studies in the literature of neuropsychology in which large amounts of brain tissue have been removed and in which not even relatively sensitive psychological tests, both in humans and in animals, have been able to detect behavioural impairment. Nevertheless, there still are individuals whose functional capacity, despite the enormous functional reserve of the brain, is close to the limits of that reserve, and who need only one further small push to produce major alterations in their ability to perform as a viable organism. These graphs simply underscore the importance of long-term, longitudinal studies of the effects of various chemical agents on performance.

The key role of longitudinal studies is also underscored by our experience with methylmercury. In Minamata, Japan, which provided the first instance of a large scale ecological threat from this substance, some health officials observed that children, now teen-agers, from the exposed families, seem to show deficits in school work and athletic ability not discerned earlier. However, these observations have not been systematized. The laboratory data, though, are even more striking. Spyker, Sparber and Goldberg (11) carried out a longitudinal study of mice exposed to methylmercury *in utero*. At the age of 3 to 4 months, mice who showed no overt neurological deficit or any other differences from controls performed in a peculiar fashion on open field and swimming tests. Much later, at 1.5 to 2 years of age, many of the mice, who never before had shown any effects of their prenatal exposure, began to display a variety of neurological signs ranging from overt postural defects to aphagia and hyperphagia (12).

When we consider that Kety's chart really begins with birth, at which time functional capacity, as defined by neuronal cell density, is 140% of what it is in the late teens, then it is easy to see why damage inflicted prenatally might not reveal its full consequences until a point in the life of the organism at which it has lost most of its reserve capacity.

These phenomena have their counterparts with psychotropic drugs. Studies by Werboff and his collaborators (13), and others, have shown that prenatal exposure to some rather common CNS drugs can produce behavioural deficits not readily apparent except by behavioural tests. Developmental pharmacologists have shown that such early exposures can also produce long-term changes in brain amines. For example, haloperidol administered to rabbit mothers during days 1-7 after parturition produces postural deformities in the nursing offspring at oral dose levels of 1 mg/kg/day (14). Even at four weeks of age, the offspring were not free of coordination dysfunctions, a process that indicates some disruption of the developing dopaminergic systems within the brain.

At the other end of the age scale, some investigators suggest that the prevalence of tardive dyskinesia among elderly patients implicates diminished CNS capacity as a predisposing factor (15, 16, 17). Alberts (18) has proposed a similar argument for the age-related onset of Parkinsonism. Consider, too, the possibility that exposure to environmental contaminants or alcohol may render an individual more susceptible to toxic effects from CNS drugs.

Finally, I must say a word about the importance of behavioural techniques in the assessment of toxicity. It is not enough simply to observe an organism if one wishes to determine precisely whether or not, and where, a deficit resides. A special concern must be focused not merely on the application of standardized behavioural techniques, but on the development of special methods that will be sensitive to changes in the constellation of effects that may be taking place over time.

SUMMARY

Both psychoactive drugs and environmental pollutants present problems in the evaluation of long-term consequences of exposure. The most prominent such consequence of major tranquilizer treatment is disorders of movement, especially the tardive dyskinesias. Administering haloperidol to a cebus monkey for a period of eight months revealed a progressive change in the response. Early in the program the monkey would be sedated 2-4 hours after drug. With time, the response altered gradually, its most striking feature the irruption of periods of violent movement, resembling convulsions. Exposure to environmental contaminants such as heavy metals (manganese, mercury), also shows a progression in the constellation of symptoms. Such progressions evoke the question of subclinical brain damage, especially arising in a gradual, insidious fashion. The brain loses reserve capacity with age under even "natural" conditions, and even small additional accelerations in loss of function can produce considerable changes in brain "age." The apparent susceptibility of elderly patients to psychoactive drug side effects and diseases such as Parkinsonism might be explained by such a phenomenon.

ACKNOWLEDGEMENTS

The preparation of this paper was supported, in part, by Grant MH-11752 from the National Institute of Mental Health, Grant GI-30097X from the RANN Program of the National Science Foundation, and in part by a contract with the U.S. Atomic Energy Commission at the University of Rochester Atomic Energy Project and has been assigned Report No. UR-3490-402.

REFERENCES

1. Crane GE: Clinical psychopharmacology in its 20th year. Science 181:124-128, 1973.
2. Ayd FJ Jr: Persistent dyskinesia: a neurologic complication of major tranquilizers. Med Sci 18: 32-40, 1967.
3. Hershon HI, Kennedy PF, McGuire RJ: Persistence of extrapyramidal disorders and psychiatric relapse after withdrawal of long-term phenothiazine therapy. Brit J Psychiat 120: 41-50, 1972.
4. Oldham AJ, Bott M: The management of excitement in a general hospital psychiatric ward by high dosage haloperidol. Acta Psychiat Scand 47: 369-376, 1971.
5. Mena I, Marin O, Fuenzalida S: Chronic manganese poisoning: clinical picture and manganese turnover. Neurology 17: 128-136, 1967.
6. Cotzias GC, Papavasiliou PS, Ginas J: Metabolic modification of Parkinson's disease and of chronic manganese poisoning. Ann Rev Med 22: 305-326, 1971.
7. Neal PA, Flinn RH, Edwards TI: Mercurialism and its control in the Felt-Hat Industry. U.S. Public Health Service, Public Health Bulletin No. 263, 1941.
8. Hartung R, Dinman B, Editors: Environmental Mercury Contamination. Ann Arbor, Ann Arbor Science Publishers, 1972.
9. Weiss B, Simon W: Quantitative perspectives on the long term toxicity of methylmercury and similar poisons. In Behavioral Toxicology. Edited by B Weiss and VG Laties. New York, Appleton-Century-Crofts (in press).
10. Kety SS: Human cerebral blood flow and oxygen consumption as related to aging. Res Publ Assn Nerv Ment Dis 35: 31, 1956.
11. Spyker JM, Sparber SB, Goldberg AM: Subtle consequences of methylmercury exposure: behavioral deviations in offspring from treated mothers. Science 177: 621-623, 1972.
12. Spyker JM, Behavioral teratology. In Behavioral Toxicology. Edited by B Weiss and VG Laties. New York, Appleton-Century-Crofts (in press).
13. Werboff J: Developmental psychopharmacology. In Principles of Psychopharmacology. Edited by WG Clark and J deGiudice. New York, Academic Press, 1970, pp 343-353.
14. Lundborg P: Abnormal ontogeny in young rabbits after chronic administration of haloperidol to the nursing mothers. Brain Res 44: 684-687, 1972.
15. Crane GE: Tardive dyskinesia in patients treated with major neuroleptics: a review of the literature. Amer J. Psychiat 124: 41-48, 1968.
16. Edward H: The significance of brain damage in persistent oral dyskinesia. Brit J. Psychiat 116: 271-275, 1970.
17. Brandon S., McCelland HA, Protheroe C: A study of facial dyskinesia in a mental hospital population. Brit J Psychiat 118: 171-184, 1971.
18. Alberts WW, Wright EW, Levin G: Threshold stimulation of the lateral thalamus and globus pallidus in the waking human. Electroenceph Clin Neurophysiol 13: 68-74, 1961.

Possible Measures to Reduce the Prevalence and Severity of Alcohol and Drug-Related Cerebral Damage

Patricia Wilkinson

A number of factors are already thought to contribute to the development of alcohol- and drug-related brain damage. Among them are age and sex (1), nutritional status (2), the presence of other toxic factors such as congeners in certain alcoholic beverages (3), and possibly also anoxia, infections and trauma. By far the most important however, is the exposure to the major toxic agent itself. Without ingestion of alcohol, cannabis, amphetamine, heroin or what you will, there would be no alcohol- or drug-related brain damage. Furthermore, the heavier the ingestion of the agent, the more likely it is that damage will occur. A number of investigations have identified a level of alcohol consumption above which there is definite risk of damage to physical health (4, 5, 6) particularly the liver and the nervous system. Similar levels of safe and unsafe consumption are less well defined for other drugs as yet, but they surely must exist.

It follows then that in any community, the incidence of brain damage will be directly related to the incidence of excessive drinking or drug consumption. Reducing the numbers of excessive drinkers or drug users will therefore reduce the incidence of cerebral damage, and other alcohol- or drug-related complications. It matters little in this context whether these excessive users can be labeled alcoholic or drug-dependent. The damage results from the degree of exposure, rather than the presence of dependence or loss of control.

Traditionally however, measures aimed at reducing or controlling problems resulting from excessive drinking have usually been directed towards alcoholism and alcoholics. Efforts have been made to identify alcoholic and pre-alcoholic traits and personalities. Normal or social drinking and levels of drinking have not come under scrutiny except by the temperance movements. As Kettil Bruun has stated (7), approaches and policies have been towards alcoholism rather than alcohol control. This is because alcoholics have been perceived as quite different from other drinkers rather than as an extreme of the normal continuum.

More recently, however, through the work of epidemiologists such as Ledermann (8), and de Lint and Schmidt (9), it has been realised that normal drinkers and alcoholics are not two distinct and separate groups. Instead, when levels of alcohol consumption in a population are studied, normal drinkers and alcoholics are found to occupy merely two different parts of a single smooth distribution curve which ranges from abstinence to very heavy drinking (Fig. 1). There is a majority, or peak, of light to moderate drinkers at one end of the curve, and a small 'tail' of drinkers at the other end who exceed a safe level of intake and among whom can be identified the alcoholics. There is no second 'alcoholic' peak as there would be if alcoholics were 'different'.

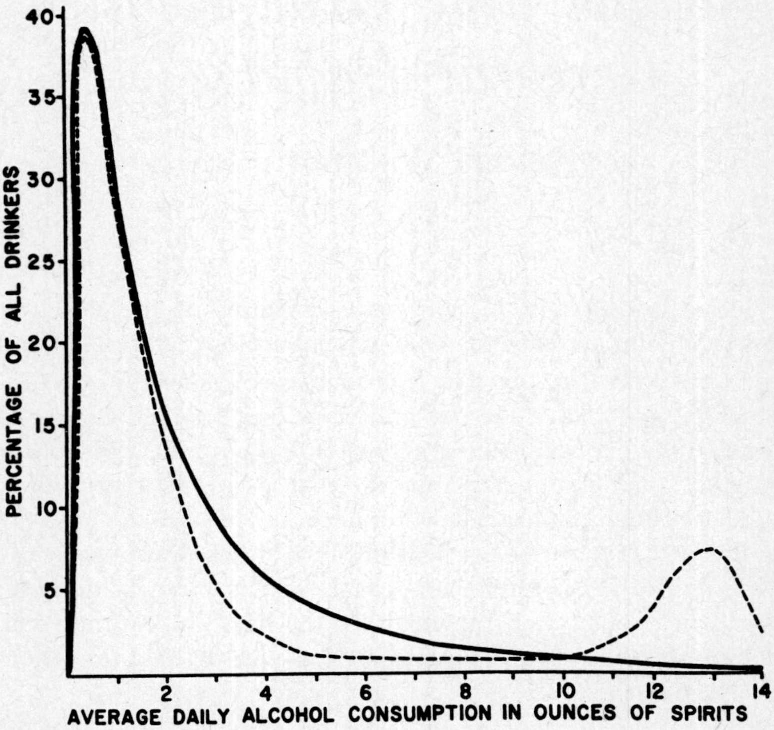

Figure 1. *Distribution curves showing the percentage of all alcohol users at each level of average daily intake of alcohol. The broken line (— — — —) shows the type of distribution of alcohol intake that would be found if alcoholics were clearly different from the rest of the population in their drinking habits. The solid line (————) shows the type of distribution that is really found.*

Furthermore, in cultures or populations where there is a high degree of acceptance of alcohol use, or where alcohol is cheap and easily obtainable, the whole distribution curve is shifted to the right. (10) Average consumption is higher and a larger number of people exceed the safe limit. Alcoholics and alcoholic complications become more common. Conversely, when alcohol use is discouraged or made difficult or expensive, the curve shifts to the left and there is a reduction in the number of heavy users exposed to the risk of toxic complications (Fig. 2).

The epidemiology of drug use is less well established, but surveys in Canada suggest that distribution curves for drug consumption resemble those found for alcohol: a majority of moderate users tailing off to a small group of very heavy users (11). If, then, easy access and social acceptance are likely to lead to relatively large numbers of heavy users and a high incidence of toxic complications, these could conceivably be reduced by making the commodity more expensive, harder to obtain or unfashionable.

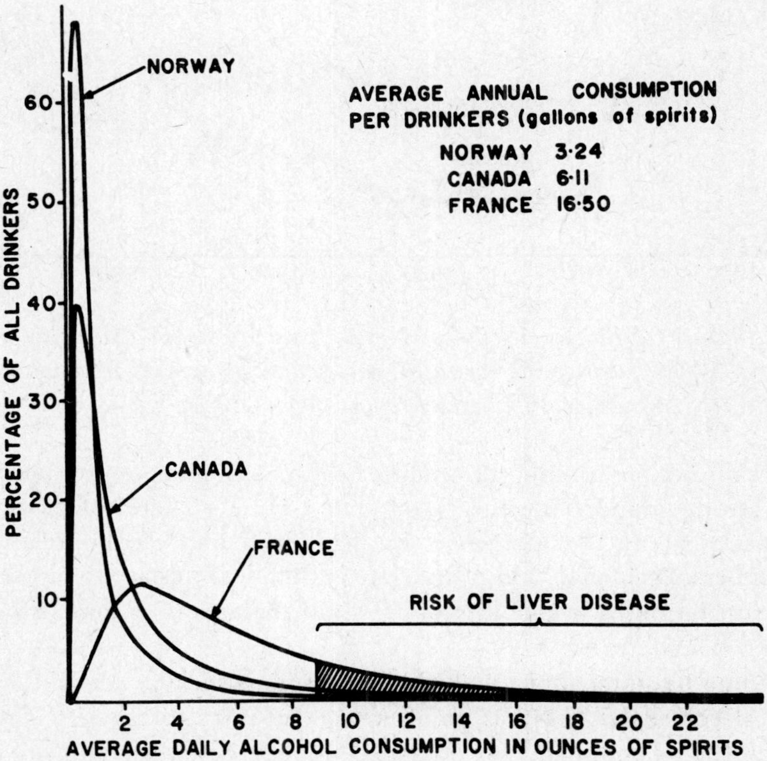

Figure 2. *Distribution curves for alcohol use in Norway, Canada and France in 1968. The higher the average* per capita *intake, the more the distribution curve shifts toward the high-intake end of the scale. The hatched area indicates the levels of intake associated with a proven risk of liver disease.*

The first measure was used in England in the eighteenth century, when gin was sixpence a bottle and drunkenness, alcoholism, cirrhosis of the liver and other alcoholic complications were rife in the cities (12). The second measure was applied in North America in this century between 1916 and 1932, the prohibition years. Both these measures worked – as far as combating alcoholism was concerned. In both situations, the average consumption of alcohol was reduced and the numbers of heavy drinkers and alcoholics decreased (12, 13). More important in the present context, the incidence of physical complications was reduced also. Klatskin showed this very clearly in his study of deaths from cirrhosis in the years before, during and after repeal of prohibition (Fig. 3). Unfortunately other social evils were unchecked – in the case of prohibition were even fostered. This does not negate the effect that

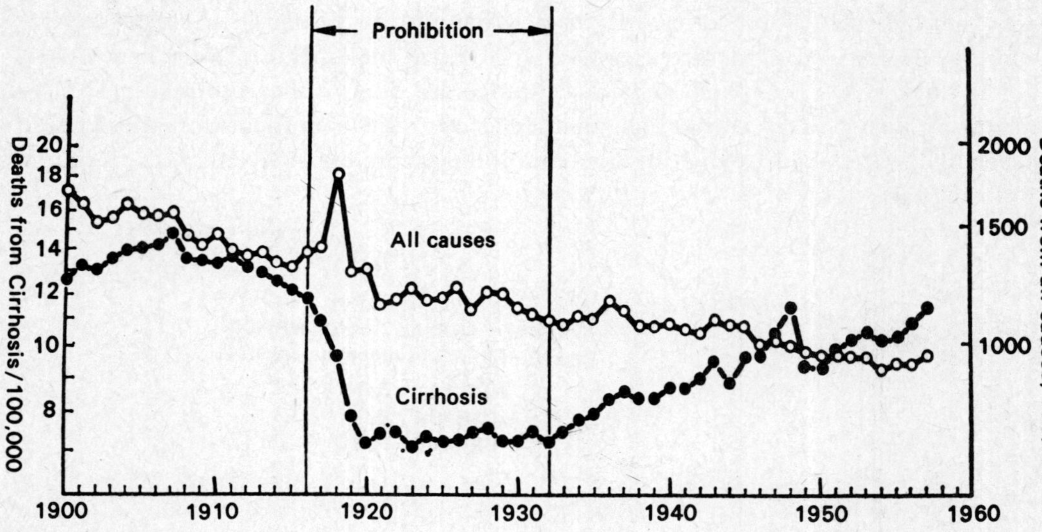

Figure 3. *Death rates from liver cirrhosis and from all other causes in the U.S.A. from 1900 to 1960. During the prohibition years there was a sharp fall in the cirrhosis death rate. Immediately after Repeal it began to rise again.*

restriction had on public drinking and public health. The changes produced by these measures are strong support for the thesis that a society's level of drinking determines to a large extent the incidence of alcoholism and alcohol-related disease among its members. If alcohol- and drug-related complications are to be reduced in a society, then restriction of availability – by legal or financial means or both – is a measure to be considered.

Can anything be done about making their use less socially acceptable, and will this have any effect? Bales (14) has pointed out that in cultures where drunkenness is not tolerated or condoned, for instance among Jews, alcoholism is a little problem. Similarly Kalant (15), quoting Chopra, commented that Indians in their own country scorn the use of cannabis, although it is not illegal. In India, there are few regular users of the drug, and very few heavy users. By contrast, westernised Indians living in a culture where cannabis is illegal but fashionable, are as prone to use and presumably mis-use it, as are the non-Indians around them.

Changes in public attitudes towards more moderate consumption and less tolerance of excessive drinking or drug use can thus be expected to produce changes in the incidence of alcohol- or drug-related disease. How can such changes be made?

Massive education compaigns have been suggested, indeed are even being mounted. Increased knowledge of the actions, pleasurable and otherwise, of the various psychoactive drugs; their effects on mental and physical function and behaviour; safe and unsafe levels of consumption; these must all help engender a more responsible attitude towards alcohol and drug use. But at the same time, there are tremendous pressures in the opposite direction, particularly in the advertising of alcoholic beverages. At present in most Western societies, massive advertising campaigns are directed at the drinker, particularly the young drinker who is still experimenting and establishing his norms. He is urged to drink more and more, stronger and stronger liquor. Strong drink is equated with sex, sin and sophistication. Standard educational programmes have little chance against these messages. Should some measures be taken against this kind of seduction, as are now being taken against cigarette advertisements?

While attempting to reduce the consumption of a community as a whole, measures directed towards detection and treatment of susceptible individuals should be ignored. No definite alcoholic, pre-alcoholic or drug-prone personality has been convincingly identified, but certain 'at risk' groups are known to exist. Children reared by alcoholic parents stand a greater than normal chance of becoming alcoholics (16). Young drug-dependent persons frequently report that their parents use large amounts of alcohol and legally obtained drugs (17). Should efforts be made to find these children and help them develop better methods of coping with life than their parents have shown to them, *before* they begin to misuse drugs themselves? This would be expensive, lengthy and demanding case work, fraught probably with legal and ethical problems, but it might be worthwhile.

Later in life, certain occupations and industries carry a special risk for the development of alcoholism. They include breweries and distilleries, the liquor sales and catering trades, the waterside, and journalism. In the past, public health measures have been instituted to protect workers from other industrial and occupational hazards. Do these trades have an obligation to provide educational, diagnostic or treatment facilities for their workers?

Since alcoholic brain damage occurs only after many years of drinking, intervention even after alcoholism has developed could help reduce the numbers who develop the complication. But if there is to be a real margin of time for treatment, the existence of a drinking problem must be recognised far earlier than it is now. At present, alcoholics rarely seek skilled help until they have been drinking excessively for many years. Among the patients studied at St. Vincent's Hospital, initial presentation came after some eighteen years of heavy drinking (18); brain damage was apparent, on average, after 23 to 26 years of heavy drinking, only five to eight years later. It is imperative then that measures be instituted which will facilitate earlier diagnosis of the alcoholic. Screening procedures such as the MAST test (19), and that compiled by the Criteria Committee of the National Council on Alcoholism (20) should help educate the medical profession to earlier diagnosis.

Unfortunately, most medical complications, certainly those classically associated with alcoholism, occur late in the natural history of the disease. Similarly with many other drug dependences, particularly to sedatives, the patient may remain physically healthy long after severe social problems have emerged. Domestic, legal or occupational problems may occur early but not be recognised as symptoms. Birrell (21) has complained of this 'compartmentalisation' of the alcoholic's life style. A man may be recognised as a dangerous driver, a wife beater, an unreliable worker; his wife may be known to be neurotic and his children to be doing badly at school, yet until he develops liver failure, alcoholism is not even thought of. As well as the medical profession, police, teachers, employers and the judiciary must be alerted to the various social indicators of alcoholism and other drug-dependent states. Drink-driving offences are at last being recognised as being suggestive of early alcoholism

(22, 23, 24). Certain work patterns have been described as pathognomonic of alcoholism (25), and these must be made more widely known to industry.

With early recognition of course, comes the need for early treatment, and the crying need in almost all countries is for more and better treatment facilities for both alcoholism and drug dependence. I will not enlarge on this except to remind you that facilities need staff. As yet, in many parts of the world staff are scarce because addiction is not a fashionable, some times not even an acceptable, specialty. At the risk of appearing cynical, I would suggest that alcoholism and drug addiction might be a more attractive area of practice if appointments carried better prospects and bigger salaries.

In considering treatment facilities, the difficult question of compulsory measures must also be debated. How far is a society entitled to interfere to protect an individual from himself? Even those countries which can use compulsion on a wide scale seem loath to do so.

Although the natural history of alcoholic brain damage is still imperfectly understood, there is evidence that its progress can be halted if drinking is stopped, and considerable return of cerebral function can be achieved. We have now observed a small number of patients who, initially quite unable to care for themselves, have, over a period of enforced abstinence, been able to return to a normal life in the community. This process of recovery is slow, and prolonged careful supervision is necessary. Few countries have a sufficient number of institutions to care for any but the most advanced of their demented alcoholics, and indeed institutions may not be the best places to encourage recovery of function. Better results might be achieved if facilities for supervised care of a patient in the community were developed. Support and guidance of the relatives who undertake the supervision, combined with day centres, home visits, sheltered workshops and short-term residential homes, might enable more patients to be treated without institutionalisation.

So far, only the major agent has been considered in the development and progression of cerebral damage in alcoholics and drug dependents. Other factors are known to affect cerebral metabolism and can contribute to the damage. The B group of vitamins, in particular thiamine, nicotinamide, folate and B_{12} are all concerned with metabolism of nervous tissue, and deficiencies of these vitamins can predispose or lead to loss of function. Heavy drinkers are particularly liable to such deficiencies anyway, because of poor nutrition, malabsorption and increased metabolic needs. In Australia, where there is a lot of heavy beer drinking, there is currently concern at evidence of subclinical thiamine depletion being found in apparently healthy people (26). Various remedies are being suggested such as improved education in eating habits, and thiamine supplementation of bread and flour, which is not compulsory at present in Australia. It has even been suggested that thiamine should be added to the beer.

When the established alcoholic is treated, vitamin stores must be replaced promptly and adequately. Care must be taken too, to avoid depleting precariously low stores further by giving large amounts of carbohydrate orally or by infusion, without generous vitamin supplements. In treating the sick alcoholic, other cerebral insults, such as anoxia from respiratory disease and amine toxicity from liver disease must be avoided. So often an alcoholic receives less than optimal medical treatment, simply because he is an alcoholic.

As yet, our knowledge of alcoholism, drug dependence and related brain damage is far from complete. Until further research fills the gaps, the best possible measures to prevent or limit these problems cannot be envisaged. In other words, further research is in itself an urgent measure. Methods of changing community attitudes need to be developed. Much work needs to be done by many professions to enable them to recognise the alcoholic earlier in his disease. By studying the criminal records of alcoholics and relating them chronologically to drinking histories, it should be possible to find patterns of offences associated with early or even prodromal alcoholism.

At present, we have no good indicator of early brain damage. Much research is needed to find more sensitive methods of recognising and quantitating loss of cerebral function. More must be discovered about the natural history of the disease process too; not only what factors initiate it and how, but how much it is reversible; and if function returns, by what means.

Finally, a most important area of research is the continuing critical evaluation of any and all measures which may be instituted, both preventive and therapeutic. Success or failure must be balanced against cost, in terms of money, time, personnel and loss of freedom to the individual.

Most of the measures suggested here involve expense, many of them also encroach on individual rights and liberties. Their implementation is the concern and responsibility not just of expert groups, but of society as a whole. Perhaps a final very important measure will be to ensure that facts, which expert groups discover, are communicated accurately to as wide a section of society as possible.

ACKNOWLEDGEMENTS

All figures are reproduced from "Drugs, Society and Personal Choice" by Kalant and Kalant (27).

REFERENCES

1. Horvath TB, Wilkinson P, Santamaria JN, et al: Dementia in alcoholics. (abstract). Aust Ann Med 18: 165, 1969
2. Victor M: Alcohol and nutritional diseases of the nervous system. JAMA 167: 65-71, 1958
3. Murphree HB: Effects of alcoholic beverages containing large and small amounts of congeners, Biochemical and Clinical Effects of Alcohol Metabolism. Edited by VM Sardesai. Springfield, Ill, Charles C Thomas, 1969, pp 259-265
4. Caroli J, Péquignot G: Enquête sur les circonstances diétetiques de la cirrhose alcoolique en France. Proceedings of World Congress on Gastroenterology. 1: 661-665, 1958
5. Lelbach WK: Leberschäden bei chronischem Alkoholismus. Acta hepatosplenologica (Stuttg) 13: 321-349, 1966
6. Rankin JG, Wilkinson P: Alcohol and tobacco consumption, The Health of a Metropolis. Edited by A Stoller, J Krupinski. Melbourne, Heinemann Educational Australia, 1971, pp 61-67
7. Bruun K: Dilemmas in drug control policy. Fifth Leonard Ball Oration. Melbourne, Victorian Foundation on Alcoholism and Drug Dependence, 1972

8. Ledermann S: Alcool, alcoolisme, acoolisation: Donnes scientifiques de caractère physiologique, économique et social, Institut National d'Etudes Demographiques, Travaux et Documents. Cahier No. 29. Paris, Presses Universitaires de France, 1956
9. De Lint J, Schmidt W: The distribution of alcohol consumption in Ontario. Quart J Stud Alc 29: 968-973, 1968
10. Popham RE, Schmidt W, de Lint J: Epidemiologic research bearing on legislative attempts to control alcohol consumption and alcohol problems. Proceedings of a Symposium on Law and Drinking Behaviour. Chapel Hill, N.C. 1970
11. Smart RG, Laforest L, Whitehead PC: The epidemiology of drug use in three Canadian cities. Addiction Research Foundation Substudy 1-7. Toronto, 1970
12. Trevelyan GM: Illustrated English Social History. Vol. 3, Harmondsworth, Penguin Books Ltd., 1964, pp 88-90
13. Klatskin G: Alcohol and its relation to liver damage. Gastroenterology 41: 443-451, 1961
14. Bales RF: Cultural differences in rates of alcoholism. Quart J Stud Alc 6: 480-499, 1946
15. Kalant H, Kalant OJ: Drugs, Society and Personal Choice. Toronto, Addiction Research Foundation, 1971, p 126
16. Rankin JG: Alcohol misuse, a family problem? Symposium – Alcoholism and the Family. St. Vincent's Hospital, Melbourne Third Summer School of Alcohol Studies. Sydney, Sandoz Australia, 1968, pp 15-28
17. Smart RG, Fejer D: Drug use among adolescents and their parents: closing the generation gap in mood modification. Addiction Research Foundation Substudy 3-7. Toronto, 1970
18. Wilkinson P, Kornaczewski A, Rankin JG, et al: Physical disease in alcoholism: initial survey of 1000 patients. Med J Aust 1: 1217-1223, 1971
19. Selzer ML: The Michigan Alcoholism Screening Test (MAST): The quest for a new diagnostic instrument. Amer J Psychiat 127: 1653-1658, 1971
20. Criteria Committee, National Council on Alcoholism: Criteria for the diagnosis of alcoholism. Amer J Psychiat 129: 127-135, 1972
21. Birrell JHW: A preliminary note on the drinking driver in Victoria, Australia, since 1966. Medicine, Science and the Law 10: 38-41 1970
22. Glatt MM: Alcoholism in "impaired" and drunken driving. Lancet 1: 161-163, 1964
23. Selzer ML, Vanosdall FE, Chapman M: Alcoholism in a problem driver group: a field test of the Michigan Alcoholism Screening Test (MAST). J Safety Res 3: 176-181, 1971
24. Raymond A: Characteristics of breathalysed drivers. Presented at the National Road Safety Symposium, Canberra, March 14-16, 1972
25. Trice HM, Belasco JA: The alcoholic and his steward: a union problem. J Occup Med 8: 481-487, 1966
26. Wood B, Penington DG: Objective measurement of thiamine status by biochemical assay in adult Australians. Med J Aust 1: 95-99, 1974
27. Kalant H, Kalant OJ: Drugs, Society and Personal Choice. Toronto, Addiction Research Foundation, 1971, pp 102, 104, 106

Alcohol and Brain Damage: Implications for the Treatment of the Individual Patient and for Alcoholism Programs

S. G. Laverty

Brain damage in relation to alcoholism is considered here in the following sequence: medical management of intoxication and withdrawal; continuing impairment and residual brain damage; restoration of function, rehabilitation and 'prosthetic environment'; control over prospective alcohol use. This sequence represents an order for the strategy of diagnostic and therapeutic procedures in alcoholism except that control over intake is a goal to be emphasised at every point. No consideration is given to other drugs of abuse although it may be seen that several general principles of treatment may apply to those also.

The alcoholic patient may present with signs of acute or chronic alcohol intoxication. Impairment of intellectual and motor functions, emotional liability, reduced perceptual acuity, fragmentation of the continuity of experience and amnesia may represent the depressed level of central nervous function temporarily induced by ethanol. In patients who have been drinking heavily, there may be a rapid alternation between the intoxicated and the withdrawal state, or symptoms of withdrawal may become acute on the cessation of drinking. Severe withdrawal sickness may delay collaboration in detailed clinical examination of the nervous system. A continuing confusional state associated with seizures or delirium tremens may delay a proper assessment of such functions as memory, for a full week. As the patient recovers from the syndrome of intoxication and withdrawal, general irritability, anorexia and sleep disturbances diminish. At this point it may be recognized for the first time that the patient is suffering from Korsakoff's syndrome and has a severe memory deficit.

Wernicke-Korsakoff syndrome resulting from thiamine deficiency (1-5) is highly reversible provided it is treated early. Thiamine should be given immediately when a patient presents who has been drinking heavily and eating poorly for more than a few days. Since the exact extent of dietary deficiency may be difficult to determine immediately, it is easier to give the vitamin to all patients presenting with problems of recent intoxication. Subjects in this state may be arrested for public intoxication and lodged in jails, or they may appear in non-medical facilities such as missions or flop-houses. Recommendations to local institutions of this kind should be made that vitamins be administered without waiting for medical advice. It has also been suggested that vitamins should be dispensed along with alcohol in bars (6). Thiamine is usually prescribed in doses of 50 mg. daily, and may be given intravenously for the first dose and instramuscularly until the patient is taking a normal diet. Other vitamins should be prescribed at the same time since the patient's diet has usually been generally deficient. Caution should be observed in the administration of glucose to patients in withdrawal since this may precipitate acute thiamine deficiency (5).

During this initial period of recovery from a bout of drinking, immediate treatment and continuing assessment are dependent on each other, and may at the same time have to be combined with negotiations to keep the patient in treatment, whether in hospital or in the care of relatives or as an out-patient. Detoxication is often supervised by non-medical staff or in the home. Where the problem is unusual or severe it requires a reasonable degree of medical skill and very good nursing care and the need for this should be taught: disseminated, for example, through the public health nurse. Further aspects of assessment and treatment may be relevant to the prevention of brain damage. Withdrawal seizures may be prevented by control of hydration. Alcohol suppresses the production of antidiuretic hormone which rebounds rapidly when withdrawal begins. This leads to overhydration which may be the most important mechanism provoking withdrawal seizures (7). The assessment of blood pH and alcohol levels should be made when depressed levels of consciousness or confusional states do not rapidly respond to the cessation of drinking or to appropriate adjustments in the level of medication. The possibility of poisoning by other drugs, or by drug interactions, or by ethanol-disulfiram interaction has to be considered at this point. Poisoning by methyl alcohol with attendant acidosis and almost inevitably serious consequences, remains a more than occasional hazard for alcoholics drinking non-beverage alcohol.

The co-existence of traumatic damage in association with alcohol intoxication must be considered. A detailed history from an informant may supply evidence which an intoxicated patient is unable to give. Careful clinical examination should be supplemented by the continued recording of vital signs. Injuries sustained in falls, accidents or fights may be masked by intoxication; subdural haemorrhage and perforating rib wounds are cases in point. When surgical treatment is called for, a control of intoxication and withdrawal symptoms must be a careful part of pre- and post-operative strategy. The sudden onset of delirium tremens usually imposes necessary delay in major interventions until it is brought under control. The expectation of the onset of severe withdrawal symptoms in the first two or three days should always be included when the best time for surgical intervention is being considered.

Not all patients present with acute problems related to alcohol intoxication. Initial presentation of the alcoholic, however, frequently calls for an assessment in which the possibility of medical illness including damage to the brain has to be investigated. Conventional methods of differential diagnosis, or the adoption of the problem-oriented record lead to formulations concerning the nature and presumed causes of cerebral damage, and hypotheses concerning the extent to which causes may interact. Treatment methods are appraised and checked for effectiveness; treatment manipulations and interventions also become part of ongoing assessment.

Diagnosis of brain damage in the alcoholic subject can be conveniently reviewed in relation to therapeutic expectations. Nutritional deficiency has already been mentioned. Cerebellar and vascular signs may be a part of the symptomatology of the Wernicke-Korsakoff syndrome and may respond to thiamine (5). Polyneuropathy may be a result only in part of thiamine deficiency and may represent deficiency of pyridoxine and pantothenic acid (5). Since it is an easy matter to prescribe the whole range of B vitamins as well as other nutritional supplements it is advisable to follow this global approach unless failure to improve is interpreted as the result of a more specific deficiency.

The management of head injuries and the control of epilepsy may claim priority in treatment. Continued impairment may result from medication legitimately prescribed or from illicit drug use on the part of the patient. Fluctuations depending on the action of the drug can usually be readily perceived by attentive staff who may be assisted by a systematic charting of behavioral patterns on a twenty-four hour basis. Diabetics who are also alcoholics may present with signs of cerebral impairment due to increased or reduced blood sugar levels: hypoglycaemia may also complicate alcoholism independently.

Ethanol has been shown to initiate agglutination of the circulating erythrocytes which in turn may damage nerve cells through annoxia, acidosis, and glucose deprivation (8, 22). In this way recent heavy drinking may increase blood viscosity and contribute to the development of cerebral vascular lesions. The use of anticoagulant therapy and vasodilating agents may prove to be a value in relation to recent ethanol ingestion, but the obvious condition of treatment is to discontinue drinking.

When the patient's physiological condition has been restored to a relatively normal state there remains the question of the presence and the extent of residual brain damage, and its potential susceptibility to further treatment. Three specific entities may be considered because of their relation to alcoholism and because they have a well-defined pathological basis. Wernicke-Korsakoff syndrome (5) may pass through a series of characteristic changes, from stupor or global confusion to the characteristic amnesic defect which may clear up slowly in response to thiamine. In the series described by Victor, Adams and Collins, recovery was incomplete in approximately 80 per cent of 245 cases followed for many years. There is little evidence that the continued administration of high doses of thiamine is of value after the first month of treatment, but it is probably advisable to maintain regular vitamin supplements indefinitely as a protective measure.

Degeneration of the corpus callosum (Marchiafava-Bignami disease) has been attributed to malnutrition and also to chronic methyl alcohol poisoning. According to Poser (9) "no satisfactory pathogenetic mechanism has been proposed to explain this rare and most peculiar condition." Diagnosis of this condition is rare in life. Discovery of characteristic defects following 'split-brain' experiments (10) has been extended to patients suffering from callosal lesions. Investigations of hemispherelateralised functions in alcoholics might result in early detection of this type of lesion.

Central pontine myelinolysis was first described by Adams, Victor and Mancall (11). Several etiological factors have been suggested including alcoholism and malnutrition, liver disease and a possible association with prolonged treatment of alcoholism. However this condition has been seldom diagnosed in life and no treatment is proposed.

The foregoing examples are localized pathological conditions related to but not directly caused by sustained alcohol intoxication. Other examples of focal brain damage, and perhaps the most common to be found in the alcoholic, are those of traumatic origin. Alcohol intoxication contributes heavily to road accidents, falls, and injuries sustained from aggressive action including gunshot wounds of the head.

Once the presence of residual brain damage of a presumably irreversible kind has been established, the value of rehabilitative treatment must be taken up. Investigation of focal brain damage has provided evidence concerning localization of function within the brain, and has led to the development of tests of these functions and their impairment. Analysis of function of impairment has been taken beyond what could be achieved in the conventional neurological examination by the use of standardized psychological testing. For example, Russell, Neuringer and Goldstein (12) describe a sequence of tests, devised as 'keys' both for the localization of function and development of pathological processes in brain damage. Some forty tests are involved from which evidence is derived of the presence and severity of brain damage, the side of lateralisation or alternatively, the presence of diffuse brain damage. However, the application of psychological testing as a diagnostic method presents problems and has been criticized by Miller (13) as follows:

> Psychologists interested in the effects of brain lesions have been largely motivated by theoretical considerations. There has been some attempt to use the knowledge attained in the diagnosis of brain pathology but since radiological and other diagnostic techniques available to the modern neurologist are much more effective, there is not much practical value in the psychologist being heavily committed to the diagnostic exercise except for a very limited range of conditions. A much more appropriate approach would be to try to apply knowledge of neuropsychological disturbances to the rehabilitation of the brain-damaged patient such as those who have suffered strokes or severe head injuries.

A more specific analysis of psychological impairment can however be valuable, not only as an aid to the diagnosis of lesions, but as a process of identifying disabilities and suggesting methods for restoration of function. For example, Warrington and Weiskrantz (14) showed that patients with characteristic Korsakoff-type amnesia could recall learned material when aided by partial information or clues. This has relevance to the anatomy of memory but has also provided a basis for practical methods to help the Korsakoff patient control his social behavior. Increasing interest has been taken in rehabilitation, particularly by the Russian neuropsychologist, A. R. Luria and his colleagues. Several publications by Luria are now available in English (15-19). Bowden (20) notes that there were four major postulates which Luria has developed. First, that the cerebral component of any functional cortical system results from the interaction of a constellation of cerebral areas. A functional system is localizable in the sense that damage to any one of the areas involved destroys the functional system, and defects result thereby. Second, a given psychological activity may be performed in different ways, that is, by different functional cortical systems. Thus, a psychological activity is not localizable in the sense that if damage to a structure destroys a functional cortical system upon which it is based, another functional system cannot be developed which would carry out that same activity. Third, the most important adaptive functions that man possesses such as abstraction, computation and speech depend upon functional cortical systems which are acquired rather than innate. The fourth major assumption is that the most important determinants of functional cortical systems in man are derived from the organization of the social environment. Various methods of restoration of function are based on the model in which new learned connections come to be established within the functional cortical system. The methods of rehabilitation which have been largely developed in the Soviet Union consist of detailed stimulus-response situations using special techniques such as the study of movement with spoken reinforcement, 'the combined motor method,' supplementing of sensation in a paralysed limb by indicators from other modalities, and techniques which promote a generalization of partial functions into more complete ones. I have no clear information on the criterion for, or the degree of recovery achieved by these methods. Some features of these techniques are undoubtably used in rehabilitation clinics in North America. One thing is clear: much effort and devotion must be put into this kind of retraining. The mobilization of relatives and friends and co-workers has been well described for the aphasic patient (21) as well as some of the techniques in use. One may wonder if the combined disability of alcohol addiction and brain damage is likely to deter this necessary and extensive support.

The capacity for restoration of function described by Luria and others is appropriate only to focal brain damage. The question is frequently raised as to what extent the clinical picture of the chronic alcoholic is contributed to by physical impairment, and to what extent this might be related to brain damage of a specific or diffuse kind. Postmortem findings in chronic alcoholics (22-24) have shown generalized shrinkage, ventricular enlargement, atrophy of cortical grey matter, perivascular hemorrhages and fat embolism. Lynch (22) has suggested that more severe damage is seen in the well-nourished alcoholic than in the poorly nourished. The effects of ethanol on blood viscosity, leading to thrombosis of small vessels, may be expected to lead to diffuse or patchy anoxic lesions (8, 22). Abnormalities of the electroencephalogram, (24, 25), radiological evidence of atrophy (26, 27), and psychological test (28, 29) results confirm evidence of brain damage in chronic alcoholics. It must be stated however that well-defined syndromes of intellectual impairment are not seen with any regularity even in the heaviest drinkers, apart from those associated with the specific clinical-pathological entities described above. If diffuse brain damage was sufficiently severe one might expect a picture similar to that of cerebral arteriosclerosis. Diagnostic difficulties may have to do with factors due to ageing, or in making the distinction between anticipated intellectual decline and that which has been hastened by drinking. Brain-damaged alcoholics may also have retreated into occupational and social situations in which defective performance remains undetected, into a life where they are not employed or responsible, such as living in a skid-row environment. However, when a number of such alcoholic patients were allowed to remain in a long-term hospital ward it was found that the majority were able to work from the ward and manage their own affairs quite well while being kept sober by the use of Antabuse. Some of the apparent deterioration of the chronic alcoholic appears to result from his ongoing drinking and social habits rather than from permanent damage. More detailed investigations are necessary to demonstrate impairment in this context, and I have no doubt that the contribution of alcohol to such damage will soon be demonstrated. It is worth noting that intellectual impairment has also been attributed to Antabuse (disulfiram) but in a controlled study no support was found for this view (31).

When medical, rehabilitative or restorative treatments have secured their best improvement, the brain-damaged patient may yet find it difficult to resume life in the general society, either as a result of defective perception, skills, or judgment; or because general behaviour is not acceptable. To help patients in this plight, suitable environments may have to be found for them either in the community or in an institution. Even the restricted life that may have to be accepted can be given interest and dignity if an interested spouse, relative or friend is prepared to accept the challenge. Institutional life can also be improved by the use of methods appropriate to each individual case, and the development of what Lindsley (32) has called "the prosthetic environment".

The presence of depressive illness should always be positively sought for in alcoholic patients. It is common and when it presents with symptoms of withdrawal, apathy or intellectual slowness, it may give the impression of impairment of the kind usually attributed to organic deficit (33). Affective disorders associated with brain damage can be separated from mood disorders of a periodic kind, and from reactive depressions; the latter varieties can more readily be treated with drugs and psychotherapeutic methods.

The presence of brain damage has implications with respect to the patient's prospective use of alcohol. Intoxication is likely to lead to increase of impairment and poor control over behaviour (34). The presence of brain damage has even been given as a reason for the development of physical addiction (35) but without convincing evidence. The brain-damaged patient is expected to have difficulty in learning and for this reason is usually excluded from therapeutic programs concerned with teaching abstinence or the control of drinking. However, the brain damage may be associated with improvement in such behaviour as described by Engel (36) in which the subject after development of Korsakoff's syndrome lost the desire to drink. Engel's patient was an intelligent, very assertive man, a business consultant employed as a free-lance trouble-shooter and notorious for his aggressive but effective way of handling company dilemmas. Always under pressure, he suffered from nervous tension and a wide variety of psychosomatic conditions including asthma and hypertension. He was also a severe alcoholic. In his early fifties, he suffered from a classical Korsakoff syndrome from which he made sufficient recovery to be able to live on a farm with his family and carry out many daily chores. His personality was quite changed. His aggressiveness, psychosomatic symptoms and interest in alcohol disappeared and for the first time in his life he appeared contented.

A reduction in alcohol consumption tends to occur after the age of fifty. One is inclined to attribute this not only to loss of tolerance and the recognition of the accumulating disadvantages of drinking, but also to a loss of drive, which may be accentuated by cerebral damage. The paradox of alcoholism is that an enjoyable habit turns into a source of misery. Renunciation is a hard lesson to learn and made easier when desires become attenuated. La Rochefoucauld has a maxim "when our vices give us up we flatter ourselves that we are giving up them" (37).

An effect of alcohol on the brain-damaged subject may be to expose impairment which is not apparent in the sober state but which may be disclosed when the subject is faced with complex tasks or is under stress.

The captain of an English ship was Swedish by birth but worked with English-speaking crews for many years in which situations he used that language alone. A symptom of his developing alcoholism was his tendency to relapse into Swedish when intoxicated, particularly after dinner, when his captive listeners would become aware that he was talking to them in a language that they could not understand. Intelligence testing showed signs of organic deficit. The captain stopped drinking and was able to continue his job for four years before retiring at the usual age. His judgment and seamanship based on many years of experience appeared to hold up, despite the gross lapses described. The patient appeared to have changed because he perceived the severity of the social consensus towards his behaviour. Such consensus is a powerful factor in rehabilitation.

When new learning is impaired, the patient may be taught to depend on external controls to improve his own behaviour. A fifty-five year old widow suffering from considerable memory deficit after one year of vitamin therapy lived with her daughter who went out to work. In her attempts to sustain conversation she had the irritating habit of asking the same question over and over again. It became difficult to find paid companions who would stay with her. Her daughter pressed for her admission to hospital for a prolonged period. As an alternative the patient was taught to use conspicuously placed wall-charts on which she or her listener wrote down topics that had already been discussed. Other written clues and instructions such as remembering to turn off the stove or light were placed in appropriate places. The patient found that she could use such instructions to herself to remember to do things, particularly when they were placed close to reinforcements such as cigarettes or sweets. Included was one instruction that she must *not* telephone for a cab driver to deliver alcoholic beverages to the house. When on holiday and without these features of her domestic environment the patient relapsed into the same habits as before.

The confabulation and difficulty in 'changing set' seen in Korsakoff's syndrome may be manipulated in therapy although the memory deficit persists. An accountant with this syndrome came into hospital during April at a time when he had been worried about completing the income tax returns of numerous clients. In hospital he had difficulty finding his way about, misidentifying the people around him, many of whom were changing from week to week. He was able however, to negotiate much better in his brother's home with the exception that he found it difficult to restrain himself from contacting former clients under the impression that their income tax should be completed immediately. Written instructions and date-checking which he carried with him proved more helpful in changing this behaviour than verbal exhortation.

The treatment of the individual brain-damaged alcoholic has to be integrated into the structure of therapeutic programs for alcoholics. Otherwise these patients are apt to be overlooked. Alcohol programs should incorporate the following policies and procedures:

1. Dietary supplements should be used routinely to prevent the deficiencies of thiamine and other vitamins. This practice should also be widely taught so that all those having to do with heavy drinkers are able to implement it at the same time as trying to persuade the alcoholic to bring his drinking under control.

2. Detailed and careful treatment for the intoxication-withdrawal syndrome should be available from practitioners generally, but also from those working in the detoxication centres or other situations where intoxicated patients may present. A control of hydration, the prevention of epilepsy and the early treatment of delirium tremens require good medical and nursing care together with efficient and rapid laboratory services.

3. The early diagnosis of brain damage may be difficult except in those cases where impairment in day-to-day functioning is already clear. Reliance on level of functioning in real life situations is the best guide to deciding in what detail the analysis of impairment should be made. The periodic checking of disability is necessary to ensure that brain damage is in fact residual and not the result of continuing active pathological changes. This requires a check by a physician, neurologist or neuropsychologist at intervals.

The provision of restorative or rehabilitive therapy for the impaired patient may be undertaken through the developing speciality of neuropsychology, but should be planned by all having to do with the patient: health care and social workers, family and community volunteers and agencies. Facilities should be developed to improve collaboration between the neurological clinic, the addiction treatment team and the neuropsychologist.

Treatment for excessive alcohol use should be initiated as early and intensively as possible. It must be acknowledged that, at present, patients with a definite diagnosis of brain damage tend to be excluded from treatment programs. Evidence of brain damage is associated with a poor prognosis for alcoholism (38) but this should not exclude them from treatment at whatever level they can derive benefit. Apart from nutritional deficiencies or traumatic injury, damage may be acquired slowly in a cumulative way. A teaching of control over excess drinking at the earliest possible age is clearly indicated and should be related to specific hazards from dangerous levels of consumption. Methods of therapy and public education whereby this might be brought about continue to be a central theme for the Addiction Research Foundation and others like it.

Collaboration and mutual education between professionals and nonprofessionals in this field could be carried out on a much more sophisticated level. Apart from the reassurance and optimism engendered by such contacts there should be a transmission of more specific ideas about treatment and prevention, and the handling of techniques which can be effectively carried out into social practices. A proper division of labour is required and should be planned for in the funding of health services.

REFERENCES

1. Wernicke C: Grundriss de Psychiatrie. Leipzig, Thelme, 1900
2. Korsakoff SS: Ejenedelnaja Klinicheskaja Gazeta. 5.6.7 1889
3. Phillips GB, Victor M, Adams RD: J Clin Invest 31: 859-871, 1952
4. Victor M, Adams RD: Am J Clin Nutr 9: 379-397, 1961
5. Victor M. Adams RD, Collins GH: The Wernicke-Korsakoff Syndrome. Philadelphia, Davis, 1971
6. Oki, G. (personal communication)
7. Knott DH, Beard JD, Wallace JA: Acute withdrawal from alcohol. Postgrad Med 42: 109-114, December 1967
8. Moskow HA, Pennington RC, Kniseley MH: Alcohol sludge and hypoxic areas of nervous system, liver and heart. Microvasc Res 1: 74, 1968
9. Poser CM: Demyelination in central nervous system. Ann N Y Acad Sci 215: 373-381, 1973
10. Sperry RW: Am Psychol 23: 723, 1968
11. Adams RD, Victor M, Mancall EL: Central pontine myelinolysis. Arch Neurol Psychiat 81: 154-172, 1959
12. Russell EW, Neuringer C, Goldstein G: Assessment of Brain Damage. New York, John Wiley & Sons, 1970
13. Miller E: Clinical Neuropsychology. London, Penguin, 1972, pp 121-122
14. Warrington EK, Weiskrantz L: Amnesic syndrome: consolidation or retrieval? Nature 228: 628, 1970
15. Luria AR: The Neuropsychological Study of Brain Lesions and Restoration of Damaged Brain Functions. In, A Handbook of Contemporary Soviet Psychology. New York, Basic Books, 1969
16. Luria AR: Traumatic Aphasia. English Edition, The Hague, Mouton, 1965
17. Luria AR: Restoration of Function After Brain Injuries. London, Pergamon Press, 1963
18. Luria AR: The Man with the Shattered World. New York, Basic Books, 1972
19. Luria AR, Tsvetkova LS: The programming activity in local brain lesions. Neuropsychologia 2: 1964
20. Bowden D: The functional system, keystone to Luria's neuropsychology. Paper delivered to American Psychological Association, New York, September, 1966
21. Griffith VE: A stroke in the family. A Manual of Home Therapy. Delacorte Press, 1970
22. Lynch MJG: Brain lesions in chronic alcoholism. AMA Arch Pathol 69: 342, 1960
23. Pennington RC, Knisely MH: Experiments aimed at separating the mechanical circulatory effects of ethanol from specific chemical effects. Ann N Y Acad Sci 215: 356-365, 1973
24. Courville CB: Effects of Alcohol on the Nervous System of Man. Los Angeles, San Lucas Press, 1955
25. Bennett AE, Doi LT, Mowrey GL: The value of electroencephalography in alcoholism. J Nerv Ment Dis 124: 27-32, 1956
26. Naitoh P: The value of electroencephalography in alcoholism. Ann N Y Acad Sci 215: 303-320, 1973
27. Skillicorn SA: Neurology 5: 527-534, 1955
28. Tumarkin B, Wilson JD, Snyder S: US Armed Forces Med J 6: 67-74, 1955
29. Hoffman H, Wefring LR: Sex and age differences in psychological symptoms of alcoholics. Psychol Reports 30: 887-889, 1972
30. Carlsson C, Claeson L, Petersson L: Psychometric signs of cerebral dysfunction in alcoholics. Br J Addict 68: 83-87, 1972
31. Payne RW, Carpenter G, Kessel N: Effect of antabuse on intellectual functioning. Dis Nerv System 26: 655-658, 1965
32. Lindsley OR: Geriatric Behavioural Prosthetics. In, New Thoughts on Old Age, Edited by Kastenbaum. New York, Springer, 1970
33. Post F: The Significance of Affective Symptoms in Old Age. O.U.P., 1962

34. Sherfey MJ: Psychopathology and Character Structure in Chronic Alcoholism. In, The Etiology of Chronic Alcoholism. Edited by O. Diethelm Springfield, Charles C. Thomas, 1955

35. Lemere F: J Clin & Exp Psychopath 17: 202-206, 1956

36. Engel G: Psychological Development in Health and Disease. Philadelphia, Saunders. 1962

37. La Rochefoucauld F duc de: Maxims. Edited by L. W. Tancock. London, Penguin, 1959

38. Mindlin DF: The characteristics of alcoholics as related to prediction of therapeutic outcome. Q J Stud Alc 20: 604-619, 1959

Index

19